New Paradigms in Healthcare

In the first two decades of this new millennium, the self-sufficiency of Evidence-Based Medicine (EBM) have begun to be questioned. The narrative version gradually assumed increasing importance as the need emerged to shift to more biologically, psychologically, socially, and existentially focused models. The terrible experience of the COVID pandemic truly revealed that EBM alone, while being a wonderful scientific philosophy and containing the physician's paternalistic approach, has its limitations: it often ignores both the patient's and physician's perspectives as persons, as human beings; it pays relentless attention to biological markers and not to the more personal, psychological, social, and anthropological ones, removing the emotions, thoughts, and desires of life, focusing on just the "measurable quality" of it.

Health Humanities, Medical Humanities and Narrative Medicine are arts intertwined with sciences that allow to broaden the mindset and approach of healthcare professionals. helping them to produce better care and more well-being.

Aim of this series is to collect "person-centered" contributions, as only a multidisciplinary and collaborative team can meet the challenge of combining the multiple aspects of human health, as well as the health of our planet, and of all the creatures that live on it, in a common effort to stop or reverse the enormous damage committed by humans during our anthropocentric era: a new paradigm of healthcare, education and learning to create a sustainable health system.

Fabrice Jotterand • Clara Bosco
Editors

Fostering Humanism in Surgery

Springer

Editors
Fabrice Jotterand
Center for Bioethics and Medical Humanities
Medical College of Wisconsin
Milwaukee, WI, USA

Faculty of Medicine
Institute for Biomedical Ethics
University of Basel
Basel, Switzerland

Clara Bosco
Postdoctoral Scholar, MacLean Center for Clinical Medical Ethics
The University of Chicago Biological Sciences
Chicago, IL, USA

General Surgery Resident
The University of Arizona
Phoenix, AZ, USA

ISSN 2731-3247 ISSN 2731-3255 (electronic)
New Paradigms in Healthcare
ISBN 978-3-031-82770-9 ISBN 978-3-031-82771-6 (eBook)
https://doi.org/10.1007/978-3-031-82771-6

This Springer imprint is published by the registered company Springer Nature Switzerland AG
The registered company address is: Gewerbestrasse 11, 6330 Cham, Switzerland

Preface

Fostering Humanism in Surgery offers an examination of the importance of humanism in surgical education and practice. As technology and the commercialization of healthcare are increasingly dictating the way of being and doing in medicine, there is an urgent need to reconsider what medical humanism can offer in sustaining the professional identity of surgeons and shaping the training of future surgeons. Bioethics, usually considered a guide for the professional identity of surgeons, is ill-suited for such a task, as it has produced a process of moral reasoning that is less interested in questions of personal and professional identity (related to moral agency, virtue, and character formation) and more devoted to principles of obligation concerning right actions and pragmatic considerations that optimize outcomes. This shift is problematic because it has marginalized the intellectual-moral foundation that can provide substantive meaning in surgical practice, encourage reflection on the role of the virtues and character formation in surgery, and offer a moral vision robust enough to guide the practice of surgery.

The *raison d'être* of this book is to challenge the philosophical assumptions of contemporary surgery: we must turn from the inclination that prioritizes bureaucracy, technologism, and the mere avoidance of suffering and death. We must turn from such medicine that demeans human beings, deforms the nature and goals of medicine, betrays the art (*techne*) of medicine, and hampers human flourishing. Such late modern ideations have not only trained many to see bodies as mere machines awaiting technological intervention, but also normalized a technologically conditioned marketplace of medicine that bureaucratizes the exchange of goods and services. Such ideations have convinced many to prioritize epistemology over ontology, knowing over being, creating a teleological disorientation that leaves surgeons at risk of not knowing how they are supposed to fulfill their professional roles as moral agents, and not knowing what the practice of surgery ought to be and become. This collection of essays provides an intellectually robust medical ethics beyond merely bioethics a vision of medicine—*qua* surgery, medical professionalism, and medical humanism reoriented toward the promotion of character development, compassionate care, and human flourishing for both patients and surgeons.

Humanistic Dimensions of Surgery

In the first chapter entitled "Building Character in Surgical Residency: How Surgeons Learn Wisdom and Humility," Zack Loveless and Kathryn J. Rowland argue that good character in surgery facilitates good clinical practice and fosters surgeon flourishing. They outline an Aristotelian approach to character development and stress the importance of several virtues in medicine, including courage, compassion, trustworthiness, wisdom, and humility. They also emphasize that character education should be integrated into residency training to counter the negative impact of the structural and cultural dimensions of the hidden curriculum. However, Loveless and Rowland stress that the cultivation of virtuous character traits during residency need not be limited to didactic sessions alone; rather, this developmental process can take various forms, from creating a culture that recognizes the importance of good character, celebrates its practice at the bedside, and surrounds residents with good role models who exemplify excellences of character.

The second chapter, "Phronesis as a Model for Surgical Education: Motorcycles, Bodies, and the Stochastic Arts," co-authored by Margot Kelly-Hedrick and Ryan M. Antiel, focuses on the nature of the practice of surgery. Surgeons are often perceived as mere technicians compared to the more intellectual roles of specialties like internal medicine or neurology. This view, which suggests that medicine is about cognitive analysis while surgery is purely about technical performance, overlooks the complexity, depth of knowledge, and humanism required in the practice of surgery. Drawing on the philosophy of Matthew Crawford, the authors argue that both surgeons and mechanics rely on *phronesis*, which is developed through experience and is essential for making appropriate decisions in contextually complex situations. This perspective underscores that surgical education must extend beyond technical proficiency to actively cultivate the moral and ethical dimensions of clinical practice, highlighting the importance of mentorship and community in the training of good surgeons.

In Chap. 3, "The Education of Surgeons in the Humanities," David L. Larson emphasizes the importance of the humanities in the training of surgeons. The author highlights the Accreditation Council for Graduate Medical Education (ACGME)'s statement that requires trainees to "adhere to ethical principles," and to embody character traits such as compassion, integrity, and respect. Although the ACGME recognizes the significance of humanistic aspects in clinical practice, Larson notes that clear pathways for incorporating the humanities into surgical training are lacking. He outlines important reasons why the humanities are important in the training of surgeons. In his view, they foster the development of professional identity and behavioral attributes, such as understanding, selflessness, compassion, and caring toward patients, while also enhancing clinical communication and observational skills.

In Chap. 4, Marie L. Fefferman, Megan K. Applewhite, and Peter Angelos examine the relevance of Principlism in surgery. In their contribution entitled "Ethical Principles in Surgery," they explore ethical decision-making in surgical practice through three distinct case studies, each accompanied by a nuanced discussion of the ethical conflicts at play and a reasoned path toward resolution. The authors use the ethical framework of Principlism, which encompasses the principles of autonomy, beneficence, non-maleficence, and justice, to analyze each case. Following each discussion, the authors provide recommendations that reflect the ethical complexities highlighted and emphasize that while Principlism serves as a useful guide, it does not dictate which principle should take precedence in any given situation. Determining the primacy of ethical principles in a given case requires careful deliberation by both the ethicist and the clinical care team.

The next chapter, entitled "Why Do We Need a Qualitative Philosophy of Surgery" and authored by Antti Huotarinen and Pia Sorto, argues that the surgical literature has properly covered traditional topics related to scientific and technical domains, questions in ethics, and the social responsibility of the profession. In their estimation, the academic literature currently lacks a philosophical perspective on the practice of surgery. While the philosophy of medicine has been an area of inquiry in philosophy, due to the unique characteristics of surgery, a distinct philosophy of surgery is needed in the literature. More specifically, a comprehensive analysis of the unique perspective of the inner world of surgeons while performing their craft is warranted. Usually, they note, the insights gained through surgical practice are shared between peers and learners. However, a more systematic approach using philosophical methods to develop a comprehensive philosophy of surgery might offer distinctive insights that will improve the practice of surgery and patient care.

Practical Considerations in the Practice of Surgery

In Chap. 6 Priya A. Rajdev and Nathaniel J. Soper discuss the implications of calling surgery an art, as suggested by the title ("The Art of Surgery"). There are many reasons to characterize surgery as a job, since it requires processes similar to those found in other professional activities. In this chapter, however, the authors challenge the notion that surgery can be reduced to just a job. In their view, the artistic essence of surgery becomes distinct through the exploration of what they call "the philosophy of craft work as artistic expression" and the "non-technical 'soft' skills" necessary for clinical practice. Soper and Rajdev examine the idea of surgery as a craft and the intricacies involved in operating on patients. Subsequently, they explore what is often referred to as soft skills (e.g., empathy, integrity, communication, etc.) and their relevance to the proper use of technical expertise in surgical practice.

Chapter 7 entitled "Applied Ethics in Surgery: What Do We Invite Patients to Trust?" and authored by Marguerite W. Spruce, Vishal G. Shelat, Kyler Squirrell, Douglas Brown, and Piroska Kopar, explores the interplay between trust, informed consent, and patient care in modern medicine. The authors emphasize trust as a cornerstone of healthcare, particularly in surgical settings where patients are vulnerable and must depend on their physicians. The chapter identifies three key relationships fundamental to building trust: between physicians and patients, among healthcare providers, and between the medical profession and society. By examining the evolution of the social contract in medicine, it highlights how societal changes and shifts in medical practice have impacted trust and ethical standards. Through three clinical case discussions, this chapter delves into pressing ethical concerns such as trust erosion, health disparities, and challenges posed by specialization and commercialization. Also focusing on trust, Andrew J. Neevel and Norman D. Hogikyan in Chap. 8, entitled "Preoperative Evaluation and Discussion: Trust as the Foundation," explore the surgeon-patient relationship, emphasizing that the preoperative evaluation is central to trust building. Using the case of Ms. M, a patient navigating emotional complexities after years of misdiagnosis, the chapter highlights the importance of tailoring care to individual values and preferences. The authors advocate for a holistic approach to surgical care that prioritizes the surgeon-patient relationship alongside technical skills. Ultimately, they argue that the essence of surgical humanism lies in the ability to guide patients through the complexities of their condition and what it means for their lives, while fostering trust and mutual understanding.

In Chap. 9, "Operating on the Critically Ill: The Need for Shared Decision-Making in a Technologically Sophisticated Healthcare Environment," Katherine Bakke delves into the challenges of surgical care for critically ill patients. The authors underscores that shared decision-making is more than collaborative effort; it entails a profound ethical responsibility to engage with patients as whole persons—biological, psychological, social, and spiritual—rather than viewing them solely as clinical cases. Surgeons must weigh technical considerations against the patient's overall "good," often navigating challenging ethical dilemmas. Dr. Bakke proposes a framework that prioritizes shared decision-making over technical feasibility. It challenges healthcare professionals to reflect on the ethical principle of "do no harm" in a more nuanced manner, recognizing that sometimes the most compassionate choice may be to refrain from an intervention even when it is technically possible.

The final chapter (Chap. 10), entitled "Social Responsibility in Surgical Practice" by Megan G. Janeway, Sheina Theodore, and Danby Kang, discusses the duty of surgeons to address health disparities and how to target the social causes of unequal access and health outcomes. A closer examination of social determinants of health among surgical patients reveals multifactorial influences—including race, ethnicity, gender, sexual orientation, and socioeconomic status—as well as systemic factors related to access, insurance policies, and geographic barriers. In light of these challenges, the authors focus specifically on surgery and the reasons why engaging the profession in social responsibility might be more difficult than expected due to the lack of educational opportunities on the topic, limited time, and institutional support. They also call for incorporating social responsibility into surgical practice through education, advocacy, and policy changes. Such paradigm change in surgery would aim at addressing health disparities through community advocacy and institutional changes.

Final Thoughts

This collection of essays features contributions from leading scholars interested in promoting humanism in surgical education and practice. It provides an overview of some of the most pressing challenges in surgery as well as potential paths to address them. We hope that this volume will benefit practitioners, learners, and scholars and enrich ongoing discussions on how to sustain the humanistic dimensions of the profession. To this end, we believe that further in-depth philosophical analysis is necessary. However, as noted above, a philosophy of surgery remains to be born. Philosophy is certainly not the only discipline participating in fostering humanism in surgery, but it is well positioned to promote thoughtful and meaningful discussions regarding the nature and goals of surgery. We believe such examination will lead to a deeper understanding of why humanism is essential to the practice of surgery.

Acknowledgments

We would like to thank and recognize the many individuals who made possible the development and publication of this book. We are grateful for their contributions, encouragement, and help. In particular, we thank our editor, Jonathan McFarland, at Springer for his guidance, support, and giving us the opportunity to put together this collection of essays. We want to acknowledge the following individuals who served as external reviewers: Lucia Bosco, Annie Friedrich, John Fulginiti, Andrew Kastenmeier, Daniel Kim, MacKenzie Landin, David Larson, Lewis Somberg. Finally, we thank our respective academic institutions and our colleagues who allowed us to work on this book.

Milwaukee, WI, USA Fabrice Jotterand
Chicago, IL, USA Clara Bosco

Contents

Part I
Foundational Issues

Chapter 1
Building Character in Surgical Residency: How Surgeons Learn Wisdom and Humility

Zachary Loveless and Kathryn J. Rowland

1.1 Introduction

It can be reasonably argued that a surgeon should be an individual of outstanding character. Character determines our responses when stressed, fatigued, and under time constraints. The grueling hours, the long lists of patients, the increasing complexity of medical problems, and the high-stakes decision-making that are part of surgical training and practice call character into action. Character shapes and is shaped by surgeons' daily interactions and activities and influences their satisfaction with the profession. While the challenges inherent in surgical training make it an opportune time to promote positive character formation, aspects of character degrade throughout training along with well-being. This chapter describes the role of good character in facilitating good surgical practice and promoting surgeon flourishing. We outline an Aristotelian model of virtue; highlight the importance of several virtues for medical practice—including courage, compassion, trustworthiness, wisdom, and humility; and suggest how character education can be integrated into residency training.

Z. Loveless (✉)
Hyde Park Institute, Chicago, IL, USA
e-mail: zloveless@hydeparkinstitute.org

K. J. Rowland
Division of Pediatric Surgery, Department of Surgery, Washington University in Saint Louis, Saint Louis, MO, USA
e-mail: rowlandk@wustl.edu

F. Jotterand, C. Bosco (eds.), *Fostering Humanism in Surgery*, New Paradigms in Healthcare, https://doi.org/10.1007/978-3-031-82771-6_1

1.2 Character Formation During Surgical Residency

The phrase "character building" can be used to describe an experience that is difficult but results in personal growth and formation. While surgical residency qualifies as difficult, rigorous, and challenging, positive character formation is anything but guaranteed. During surgical residency, little, if any, time is devoted to intentional cultivation of trainees' character. Instead, resident character is shaped by the structure and culture of the "hidden curriculum" in medicine, which is largely negative and based upon hierarchy, privilege, vulnerability, dehumanization, and navigation and negotiation [1]. As a result of medical training, physicians decline in empathy and moral judgment and have increased rates of burnout and depression [2]. The picture that emerges is that medical education is a period of character deformation rather than positive character formation.

1.2.1 Burnout, Moral Injury, and Human Flourishing: Defining the Problem

Burnout is a syndrome resulting from chronic workplace stress and manifested by heightened feelings of exhaustion, increased mental distance from one's job, and reduced professional efficacy. Among physicians, 38–54% report being burned out, and only 43% would recommend a career in medicine to their children [3, 4]. For surgeons, despite relatively high levels of professional fulfillment, burnout rates remain high and have devastating consequences [5]. Professionally, burnout increases medical errors, depersonalization, and emotional exhaustion and decreases compassion and interaction with patients [3, 6]. Personally, burnout is associated with substance abuse, strained personal relations, depression, and suicide [7, 8].

Encouragingly, the overwhelming majority of surgical residents report that they really care about their patients and getting a tremendous amount of satisfaction from working with them [12]. Yet residents are not spared from burnout. Approximately 40% of general surgery residents meet criteria for burnout, and over 50% of general surgery residents have high levels of emotional exhaustion and depersonalization [10–13]. In fact, burnout occurs very early in resident training. In one study, 4.3% of internal medicine residents met the criteria for burnout at the start of their intern year. By the end of their intern year, 55.3% had met the criteria for burnout [9].

It is dangerous to label a physician with burnout, since it suggests that if one were to work harder to become more balanced and resilient, burnout would subside. Surgeons tend to self-select as individuals who do not shy away from hard work to become the best. If told that they need to participate in additional wellness initiatives outside of work to care for themselves and recharge for the next day, surgeons will accept the insinuation that burnout is the result of their own personal deficiency and rise to the challenge. To acknowledge that the source of the problem is not a broken individual but a broken healthcare system, the term "moral injury" has gained popularity. Moral injury refers to the challenge of simultaneously knowing the care a patient needs but being prevented from delivering that care by constraints outside an individual physician's control [14].

The challenges in the delivery of modern healthcare at a systems level are staggering. Electronic medical records and documentation requirements for reimbursement keep physicians tied to computer screens instead of spending face-to-face time with patients. Declining reimbursement means more patients must be seen over the course of the day to maintain reimbursement. As a result, each patient gets less time with the physician. In academia, this means physicians have less time to teach and mentor because teaching is not a reimbursable activity. In the face of declining reimbursements, many physicians who were formerly in private practice and many young physicians finishing training opt to join organizations as employed physicians. But even this doesn't alleviate the economic pressures and leaves physicians under the scrutiny of an ever-growing number of administrators. Add this to the burden of caring for increasingly complex patients with multiple comorbidities and attention to physician metrics based largely upon patient satisfaction instead of the objective quality of care provided. The system is not set up for good doctors to succeed.

Further, physicians are largely intrinsically motivated to pursue a career in medicine, i.e., they are moved by the inherent satisfaction with the activities that are part of medical practice [36]. Among physicians, intrinsic motivators such as sense of calling and personally rewarding hours per day were most strongly associated with high life meaning, commitment to direct patient care, and career satisfaction—indicators of low levels or absence of burnout [15]. Being extrinsically motivated—i.e., driven to perform an action for the separable outcome it will produce, like income—however, is not associated with meaning or commitment [15, 36]. Yet, healthcare delivery has devolved into a system driven by extrinsic motivation. It is no wonder that physicians face moral injury and burnout.

Human flourishing provides an apt model for understanding the state of today's physicians. Flourishing is related to, yet more robust than, well-being. Conceptions of well-being focus on psychological aspects of a person's life being good, whereas flourishing describes a state in which all aspects of a person's life are good—psychological as well as physical, social, and spiritual [16]. For instance, most accounts of well-being do not factor in the impact of a person's health or the community in which they live. Yet one cannot fully flourish if in poor health or living in a community marked by continual threats to physical safety [16]. Burnout not only impacts psychological well-being; it impacts overall flourishing, for burnout is associated with poor social and physical well-being as well. Consistent with statistics about resident burnout, when surveyed, residents score lower on flourishing indexes than established population norms [23].

The most prominent conception of flourishing analyzes it in terms of six domains: happiness and life satisfaction, physical and mental well-being, meaning and purpose, character and virtue, close social relationships, and financial and material security. Further, four pathways that lead to flourishing within each domain have been proposed: family, work, education, and religious community [22]. The four pathways are neither exhaustive nor jointly necessary for flourishing. Yet each has potentially significant effects on it. The work pathway is of particular interest in connection with burnout. It is true that physicians need to take care of themselves outside of work—to invest in personal relationships and attend to their health through diet, exercise, and adequate sleep. But it is what happens inside the hospital—caring for patients and treating illness—that makes physicians devote their lives to a career in medicine. There is much joy in being a doctor, and this does not come from what happens outside of work but from the work itself. Flourishing allows an avenue to acknowledge that work and personal life are all one's life, and both need to be good, not so much balanced, if one is to fully live well.

1.2.2 Aristotle's Virtue Theory and Character Cultivation for Flourishing

Surgical training hinders ethical conduct, and it erodes physician wellness. Here we describe what might be gained by attention to virtue development during surgical training. For virtue is thought to engender good conduct and flourishing.

In contrast to deontological theories that focus on which duties to fulfill or consequentialist theories that focus on which outcomes to promote, virtue-based theories focus on the character traits needed to act well and the kind of person one should become. The framework we adopt belongs in the tradition that begins with Aristotle—arguably the most prominent and durable conception of virtue at least in the Western tradition—and continues in contemporary philosophy and psychology [41, 42].

One's character, according to this framework, is a collection of stable and enduring dispositions that shape how one characteristically thinks, feels, and acts. A virtue is a disposition enabling us to respond admirably and excellently in some characteristic domain of human affairs. In contrast, vices are dispositions to respond poorly and maladaptively. We need virtues where some common temptation or obstacle makes responding admirably difficult. As Michael Lamb describes it, character is "especially important in helping us maintain constancy in the face of contingencies, ensuring that we stay true to our guiding values and purposes when outside events or pressures tempt us to abandon what we hold most dear [25]." For instance, it is easier to avoid what we fear or circumstances that are unpleasant than it is to endure them. Yet developing courage readies one to stand firm in fearful, risky, or painful situations where an important good is at stake—e.g., continuing to provide patient care while exposing oneself to a deadly infectious disease.

Dispositions of character are stable though not fixed aspects of one's personality. They are malleable, as the waning of empathy during medical training attests. While one may have an innate disposition for particular virtues (or vices), most of our dispositions of character fall between the extremes of virtue and vice. The goal of intentional efforts to cultivate character is to move our dispositions closer to the ideal of virtue, making our admirable responses more stable especially when faced with the circumstances that make such responses difficult. What recommends virtue over other ethical approaches is that it offers promise in helping physicians live up to the ethical standard of the profession, boosting flourishing, and ameliorating burnout.

As we demonstrate below, both physicians and patients recognize that being a good physician requires meeting various ethical demands. This is implied in the nature of the profession which aims to serve others. Of course, one may argue that ethical behavior in medicine should be informed and guided by foundational principles—like the four fundamental principles of bioethics. Yet even if these principles are accurate and essential, they need to be supported by virtuous habits.

First, it is questionable that any set of principles will cover every situation or give a sensible answer when applied to them [49, 50]. The law, e.g., is a set of principles that provides direction about what to do, is refined by experience, and is ostensibly just in the abstract. Yet laws continually run up against situations where their recommendations seem unjust [53, 54]. Second, one's character can shape how one applies these principles and one's perception of the situation to which they are applied. Suppose a physician who is arrogant, and thinks they always knows best, dismisses input from patients, their families, and the care team. They will lack information that is crucial to diagnosing and treating the patient much less information needed to tailor treatment to a patient's goals and situation. Good principles won't save us from lack of humility. In many cases physicians face, even if some consideration of the principles *would* recommend a sensible course of action, there is no time to think through what the principles recommend to do. When a physician unexpectedly encounters an upset patient or has to navigate a conflict with a colleague, their response will default to the ways they tend to respond to frustration and conflict, i.e., to their character. Third, relying on principles during deliberation may improve moral reasoning, but sound moral reasoning does not issue in sound moral action [55]. Even when we know what our principles recommend doing in a situation, we often do not follow through because it is our character, not our reasoning, that determines our reactions when we are overworked, stressed, tired, and hungry.

Further, on an Aristotelian view, acting ethically and well-being are conceptually linked. Virtues enable us to be good to others and to do well for ourselves. Thus by cultivating virtue, one is more likely to act in morally upstanding ways and, thereby, to flourish. This conceptual link is rooted in the idea that a person needs virtues to effectively navigate temptations, obstacles, and difficulties humans inevitably face. In the pursuit of any large undertaking—like getting a medical degree—one will face adversity and setbacks one must overcome and will have to forgo some pleasures now for pleasures in the future. So anyone, and especially those pursuing medicine, needs self-regulation and perseverance. By the same token, one who cannot endure any risky, dangerous, or painful circumstance will have a more difficult time than one who has the will and ability to endure them. Empirical evidence supports this connection. In one longitudinal study of flourishing, one question representing the character and virtue domain—"I always act to promote good in all circumstances, even in difficult and challenging situations"—had the most robust association with subsequent overall flourishing. Other studies show that improvements in virtue are connected [24] with improvements in nearly every domain of flourishing—increasing life-satisfaction, subjective well-being, and purpose in life, fostering better relationships and mental and physical health, and facilitating one's ability to deal with stress and adversity [17–21, 39].

1.3 The Character of a Good Surgeon

Being a good surgeon requires more than good technical skills. Technical skill and problem-solving are important, yet they should not come at the expense of being caring, reliable, and trustworthy. The nature of the physician-patient relationship, the inherent vulnerability of the patient, and the promise of the doctor to heal implicate the need for virtues on top of technical competence [37, 38]. Both patients and physicians understand that good medical practice depends on good character.

Patients describe their ideal doctor as one who is confident, empathetic, humane, personal, forthright, respectful, and thorough [28]. Sadly, patients' perceptions of physicians have become far from favorable. Only 57% of Americans believed their doctor cared about the patient's best interest all or most of the time, and only 12% thought their doctor could admit a mistake and take responsibility [26]. One study demonstrated that patients rated artificial intelligence chatbot responses as higher inquality and more empathetic than that of actual physicians [27]. Anecdotally, one author (KR) cared for a child during fellowship who had undergone over 200 operations during a 10-year span. His family was all too familiar with the medical system. Before graduation, his mother commented, "We have met many doctors that are very smart. And many that are very nice. We know that you will be a great doctor because you are both smart and nice – that is very rare."

In a UK study, experienced physicians, medical students, and premedical undergraduates agreed that a good doctor needs fairness, honesty, kindness, leadership, teamwork, and good judgment [29]. In a US sample, the majority of medical students disagreed that one could be a good physician if not a good person [35].

There is a demand to help our future physicians develop not only the medical knowledge they need but also the character traits required to succeed in medicine. In a specialty where the hours are long, the stakes are high, and cases are increasingly complex, a good surgeon needs courage, compassion, trustworthiness, wisdom, and humility. Below, we describe each of these virtues, as well as their importance for the practice of medicine, in more detail.

1.3.1 Courage

Courage is the strength to do what is right in the face of danger, risk, pain, or uncertainty. Surgeons draw on courage when they persevere through a long or complex operation and scrub in again after a surgical mistake harms a patient. They need courage to frankly share information that risks frustrating or devastating patients and their families—whether a poor prognosis, surgical complication, or medical error. Courage does not require one to face every risk or danger. On this conception, courage is opposed to recklessness as well as to cowardice. It is no sign of courage to proceed with surgery when there is great risk of complication or death with little benefit for the patient or without the skills or planning to appropriately carry out the procedure. Courage does require that surgeons not avoid situations simply because there is discomfort and danger involved, for surgeons need to be ready to act in the face of hemorrhage, trauma, and life-threatening emergencies.

1.3.2 Compassion

Compassion is fundamental to caring for those who are sick. Compassion—literally to suffer with—includes recognition of another's suffering, emotionally resonating with the suffering, and being motivated to alleviate it [56, 57]. Surgeons are trained to have the technical skills needed to relieve physical suffering. By developing compassion, surgeons can better understand their patients, improve diagnosis [40, 41], and tailor a course of treatment to a patient's situation [37] so that their technical skills are effectively deployed. Further, for many patients, suffering is more than purely physical, and not all suffering can be relieved. It is important for surgeons to be able to recognize a patient's suffering, be present with a patient in their suffering, and act as possible to mitigate some of their patient's suffering, even when there is no operation to relieve it.

1.3.3 Trustworthiness

Trustworthiness, while more a quality dependent on virtue than a virtue itself, is crucial for supporting the physician-patient relationship. The physician-patient relationship is founded on an implicit promise to help those who seek care [37]. Surgeons often meet patients when they are vulnerable, weak, and easily exploitable. To openly disclose their symptoms, to consent to surgery, to follow through with treatment, and to feel satisfaction with their care, patients must trust a physician's skill and commitment to their care [38]. Establishing trustworthiness requires honesty—so that patients can have accurate information to make informed choices and to evaluate delivery of their care. Trustworthiness also requires integrity, keeping one's deep commitments even when there are risks to social standing or well-being. Integrity is shown in classifying a case as emergent instead of elective, even though that will mean getting less sleep; in redoing the skin closure after a long procedure because it isn't quite right; and in doing what is right when no one is looking.

1.3.4 Wisdom

Practical wisdom is excellence in practical judgment—judgment of what to do. It is shown in thoughtful decision-making and insightful advice and is guided by moral aspirations, aiming at common good [53]. In the context of medicine, wisdom implies sound clinical judgment which integrates patient goals of care and is oriented by ethical concerns [58]. Surgical wisdom is not based upon the number of relative value units generated, one's technical skill, number of publications, or lines on curriculum vitae. Nor is wisdom solely based on a surgeon's clinical acumen or positions of leadership. Indeed, practical wisdom has a complicated relationship to intelligence [48]. Instead, wisdom depends on noticing and appropriately weighing relevant information; viewing treatment options from different perspectives, e.g., that of the care team as well the patient or their family; balancing these different perspectives; and on tailoring decisions to the specific circumstances of a patient's illness and situation.

1.3.5 Humility

While all the above character strengths are likely recognized as important for being a good surgeon, humility may not be regarded as important or as a virtue at all. Surgeons are not trained to be humble. They are trained to prize their skills and problem-solving abilities, whereas humility is associated with lack of feelings of superiority or arrogance [30]. Humility, moreover, is often associated with weakness and having a low opinion of oneself [31]. Yet, as C.S. Lewis quipped, "humility isn't thinking less of oneself, it is thinking of oneself less." Humility derives from the Latin *humilitas*, meaning grounded or from the earth and indicating a tendency to keep abilities, accomplishments, and strengths in perspective not to systematically devalue them. Humility, like courage, hits a mean between a vice of excess—i.e., arrogance, a tendency to overestimate or inflate one's importance, worth, or abilities—and a vice of deficiency—i.e., self-deprecation, a tendency to underestimate one's worth or abilities.

For physicians, humility includes accurate assessment of abilities, recognition of limitations, appreciation of others, and acknowledging that one is part of, and dependent on, a larger team and system, all of which foster a culture of continuous learning, collaboration, and patient-centered care [31, 32]. Humility does not mean surgeons should embrace mediocrity or incompetence. Rather, it requires acknowledging areas of weakness, admitting mistakes, seeking honest feedback, and listening to the input of others [33]. A humble surgeon is one who is confident in their technical abilities, recognizes the limits of their expertise and experience, acknowledges that their outcomes depend on a team approach, expresses gratitude for all those who participate in a patient's care, and recognizes that patient preferences, support, and social considerations are important factors in care.

1.4 Application of Character Education in Medical Education: Teaching and Cultivating Character

Good character benefits both physicians and patients. It may ameliorate burnout. Trainees appreciate the importance of developing good character to being a good physician and surgeon. Residents do not agree that to be a good surgeon you must give up sensitivity, nor are they unhappy with the personality that they must have to become a good surgeon [12]. Similarly, 72% of medical students agreed that medical educators are responsible for training students to develop good character, and they were receptive, regardless of demographic or religious characteristics, to character development in medical education [35].

Yet can virtue be intentionally cultivated? If so, how? At the University of Chicago, we have developed and implemented a curriculum since 2017 to promote character formation in premedical undergraduate students and in preclinical medical students. The Scholars in Ethics and Medicine program helps future physicians develop character strengths they need to flourish in medicine and in life by fostering engagement with exemplars, discussions that deepen understanding of virtue, and reflection on experience all within a supportive community [34, 45].

During the yearlong, for-credit program, we introduce students to an Aristotelian framework of virtue applied to medical practice; connect them with exemplar physicians who share their experience navigating difficult situations, what they learned from them, and the virtues that prepare them for similar situations in the future; pair them with early career mentors to discuss the challenges on their horizon; create opportunities for them to grow closer to their peers, mentors, and program leaders; and provide them space and time for critical reflection. Our unpublished data suggest that participants significantly increase in wisdom, epistemic humility, compassion, purpose, and psychological well-being, while peer students not enrolled in the program show declines across these measures.

Several studies support our findings that character can be intentionally developed or strengthened through targeted intervention [51, 52]. In particular, several studies show that character can be developed during one's time in university and after [44, 46, 47].

In addition, models of character education have been developed alongside these studies to guide efforts to implement character-focused curricula [34, 43, 45].

Note that intentional efforts to promote character development need not exclusively, or perhaps primarily, consist in direct instruction or *teaching* of character, e.g., by providing knowledge of when a virtue is called for or practices for developing it. Character can be taught, but it is also caught and sought [43]. That is, first, character can be caught or learned from one's environment and the influence of others. That character can be caught is implicit in the idea that the hidden curriculum of medicine explains declines in empathy and moral judgment. Positive character development thrives in an environment where people are supported, where others value good character, and where good character is routinely exhibited. Second, character development must ultimately be sought. Much like developing a skill, character development is difficult and slow-going and requires personal effort and commitment [41]. The choices made day in and day out will shape a person's character. While individuals must take responsibility for their character, efforts to educate character should strive to create an environment that motivates and provides opportunities for seeking character development [42].

The challenge for any curricular developments for surgical residents is capturing their time and allowing adequate space for reflection. Surgical residents are often too busy to eat, much less to purposefully reflect on and cultivate their character. Work hour restrictions, sicker patients, larger patient loads, and an increasing shift mentality have challenged the apprenticeship model of surgical training and undermined the community that spontaneously formed among residents and other team members. In spite of this, the need for intentional character investment is crucial. Surgical residents need opportunities and a community that will promote positive character development. Without it, both patients and residents suffer.

How might character be cultivated in surgical residency? Here we recommend some strategies for integrating character development into surgical training.

1.4.1 Create a Culture That Recognizes and Celebrates Character

To counteract the culture of medicine that leads to the deformation of character, surgical departments must demonstrate that character is valued at all levels, from leadership and faculty to residents and medical students. Departments may signal the importance of character by first articulating and celebrating a set of core virtues, like those specified above. Indeed, the importance of many character strengths is indicated in institutional statements of core values. For instance, UChicago Medicine's statement of values mentions embracing curiosity by staying open to new ideas and championing diverse perspectives, thus signaling the importance not only of curiosity but also open-mindedness and humility. Articulating the virtues of focus will set clear standards for good surgical practice and foster a consensual understanding of these norms and how they are to be realized.

But the importance of these virtues needs to be reinforced in practice, not simply in statements posted throughout the hospital. Feedback on resident performance should extend to concerns of character, e.g., how a resident listens and responds to patients, reacts to disagreement, etc. Morbidity and mortality conferences can be used as opportunities to cultivate humility, accept responsibility, and discuss trustworthiness, justice, and attentiveness. Department-sponsored talks can be devoted to discussing ethical challenges in surgical care or practices that promote virtue. Overall, the department must demonstrate the value it places on good character development.

1.4.2 Establish an Atmosphere of Friendship

Character development is stunted in isolation and benefits from a community that is mutually supportive and encouraging. Such a community is founded on friendship since friendship involves relationships of understanding, care, and mutual betterment.

With the nature of resident work hours—increasing shift work, cross coverage plans, and short rotations spent interacting with a wide number of faculty—apprenticeship models have largely disappeared from surgical resident training programs. The down time in the hospital that provided spontaneous opportunities for building community, whether during a brief lull in an overnight call or the time between cases, has been taken up by greater administrative and charting tasks and higher patient loads of increasing acuity. This negatively affects both the relationships that form between faculty surgeons and residents as well as the relationships and community between residents. As a result, the need to foster an atmosphere of friendship to have residents feel known and supported is increasingly important.

The relationship of a faculty surgeon to a surgical resident is often described as a mentor to mentee, which acknowledges the professional skills and knowledge the surgeon tries to impart to the resident, as well as the insight provided into navigating surgical practice and life as a surgeon more generally. Each aspect of surgeon mentorship benefits from creating a friendly environment among surgeons and residents, for this creates an atmosphere of trust where issues and feedback can be frankly discussed. Surgical departments can provide opportunities and space for residents and surgeons to gather informally. Surgeons can cultivate community and friendship by giving residents their attention, by showing genuine interest in the life of the resident in and out of the hospital, sharing their own story, demonstrating vulnerability, and making space for open discussion. Whether it be from chatting before a case, taking a break for coffee, or hosting dinner for the residents, these investments in time are worthwhile. It is important to consider friendship, in addition to teaching and mentorship, in training surgical residents.

1.4.3 Provide Perspective and Experience

Faculty surgeons are further along the life path that surgical residents are on. They have gone through the same situations and had the same experiences. Thus they have knowledge to share about diagnosis and treatment and also insight about the ethical dimensions of surgical life. When instructing residents, faculty may describe how to perform a procedure, what to watch out for when performed, and provide feedback on a resident's performance of it. Just the same, they can walk their residents through their thought process when having a difficult conversation with a patient or staying engaged and compassionate when under the pressure of an unending workload. If a resident makes an error, faculty can walk residents through the steps that led to it and the steps to fix it, and they can share their experiences making medical errors and how they moved on from them. How do you maintain motivation and meaning when faced with a never-ending scut list? How do you continue to show compassion when patients are rude or don't seem to care about their health? It is important to expose surgical trainees to both the good and the bad in being a surgeon. This involves demonstrating vulnerability and a willingness to be open and honest with residents and discussing challenges encountered, how to ideally navigate them, and practices that can prepare one to meet them in the future.

1.4.4 Model Good Habits

A commitment to character development must be reinforced by faculty and staff modeling the habits they hope to promote. Without that, any claims about character's importance will feel hollow. Implementing some of the strategies above already involve modeling virtuous habits. By fostering an atmosphere of friendship, one will already model humility and compassion, for example. Yet character is always on display—in the operating room, rounding on the ward, in the clinic, and in one's daily interactions with patients, peers, and trainees, for good and bad as the hidden curriculum shows. To create an environment where good character is caught, the daily activities of surgeons need to show humility, compassion, integrity, and wisdom. How do you respond to a mistake? How do you respond to input from others? How do you treat the rest of the care team? All will matter for modeling humility. This does not mean surgeons should be perfect or never make mistakes. But how to deal with fallibility and failure well is something one can model too, showing humility and integrity.

1.5 Conclusions

Although surgeons have a high sense of professional fulfillment, burnout and emotional exhaustion manifest early in surgical training and often persist through one's career. In surgical training the hours are long, the amount of clinical knowledge to master is extensive, and a mistake can result in patient morbidity or mortality. To meet these challenges while providing excellent care, a surgeon needs courage, compassion, trustworthiness, wisdom, and humility. But one does not have the character traits of a good surgeon just because one needs them, has completed residency, or even because one has them to some innate degree before entering medical school. One has the character traits of a good surgeon because they have been modeled, cultivated, and refined over time. Currently, little to no time is devoted to the cultivation of these character traits. It is of utmost importance to purposefully invest the time and attention necessary to cultivate character traits that will allow surgical residents to flourish professionally and personally.

References

1. Mackin R, et al. The hidden curriculum: a good thing? Cureus. 2019;11(12):e6305.
2. Neumann M, et al. Empathy decline and its reasons: a systematic review of studies with medical students and residents. Acad Med. 2011;86(8):996–1009.
3. Shanafelt TD, et al. Changes in burnout and satisfaction with work-life integration in physicians and the general US working population between 2011 and 2020. Mayo Clin Proc. 2022;97(3):491–506.
4. 2022 Physician Report. Medical Economics, 2022.
5. Ligibel JA, et al. Well-being parameters and intention to leave current institution among academic physicians. JAMA Netw Open. 2023;6(12):e2347894.
6. Dyrbye LN, et al. Relationship between work-home conflicts and burnout among American surgeons: a comparison by sex. Arch Surg. 2011;146(2):211–7.
7. Oreskovich MR, et al. Prevalence of alcohol use disorders among American surgeons. Arch Surg. 2012;147(2):168–74.
8. Shanafelt TD, et al. Special report: suicidal ideation among American surgeons. Arch Surg. 2011;146(1):54–62.
9. Rosen IM, et al. Evolution of sleep quantity, sleep deprivation, mood disturbances, empathy, and burnout among interns. Acad Med. 2006;81(1):82–5.
10. Rodrigues H, et al. Burnout syndrome among medical residents: a systematic review and meta-analysis. PLoS One. 2018;13(11):e0206840.
11. Martini S, et al. Burnout comparison among residents in different medical specialties. Acad Psychiatry. 2004;28(3):240–2.
12. Yeo H, et al. Attitudes, training experiences, and professional expectations of US general surgery residents: a national survey. JAMA. 2009;302(12):1301–8.
13. Elmore LC, et al. National survey of burnout among US general surgery residents. J Am Coll Surg. 2016;223(3):440–51.
14. Dean W, Talbot S, Dean A. Reframing clinician distress: moral injury not burnout. Fed Pract. 2019;36(9):400–2.
15. Tak HJ, Curlin FA, Yoon JD. Association of intrinsic motivating factors and markers of physician well-being: a national physician survey. J Gen Intern Med. 2017;32(7):739–46.

16. VanderWeele TJ, Lomas T. Terminology and the well-being literature. Affect Sci. 2023;4(1):36–40.
17. Algoe SB, Haidt J, Gable SL. Beyond reciprocity: gratitude and relationships in everyday life. Emotion. 2008;8(3):425–9.
18. Mischel W, Shoda Y, Rodriguez MI. Delay of gratification in children. Science. 1989;244(4907):933–8.
19. Moffitt TE, et al. A gradient of childhood self-control predicts health, wealth, and public safety. Proc Natl Acad Sci USA. 2011;108(7):2693–8.
20. Jeste DV, Lee EE. The emerging empirical science of wisdom: definition, measurement, neurobiology, longevity, and interventions. Harv Rev Psychiatry. 2019;27(3):127–40.
21. Fagley NS. Appreciation uniquely predicts life satisfaction above demographics, the Big 5 personality factors, and gratitude. Personal Individ Differ. 2012;53(1):59–63.
22. VanderWeele TJ. On the promotion of human flourishing. Proc Natl Acad Sci USA. 2017;114(31):8148–56.
23. Kelly-Hedrick M, et al. Measuring flourishing among internal medicine and psychiatry residents. J Grad Med Educ. 2020;12(3):312–9.
24. Chen Y, et al. Longitudinal associations between domains of flourishing. Sci Rep. 2022;12(1):2740.
25. David Henreckson ML. Character in crisis: the challenges of moral formation in higher education. Commentary 2021 https://comment.org/character-in-crisis-the-challenges-of-moral-formation-in-higher-education/
26. Funk C, Hefferon M, Kennedy B, Johnson C. Trust and mistrust in Americans' views of scientific experts. Pew Research Center; 2019. https://www.pewresearch.org/science/2019/08/02/trust-and-mistrust-in-americans-views-of-scientific-experts/
27. Ayers JW, et al. Comparing physician and artificial intelligence chatbot responses to patient questions posted to a public social media forum. JAMA Intern Med. 2023;183(6):589–96.
28. Bendapudi NM, et al. Patients' perspectives on ideal physician behaviors. Mayo Clin Proc. 2006;81(3):338–44.
29. Kotzee B, Ignatowicz A, Thomas H. Virtue in medical practice: an exploratory study. HEC Forum. 2017;29(1):1–19.
30. Toledo-Pereyra LH. Humility. J Investig Surg. 2007;20(2):63–5.
31. Tangney J. Humility: theoretical perspectives, empirical findings and directions for future research. J Soc Clin Psychol. 2000;19:70.
32. Michalec B, Cuddy MM, Felix K, Gur-Arie R, Tilburt JC, Hafferty FW. Positioning humility within healthcare delivery – from doctors' and nurses' perspectives. Human Factors in Healthcare. 2024;5:100061.
33. Reynolds CW, et al. Humility: a revised definition and techniques for integration into surgical education. J Am Coll Surg. 2023;236(6):1261–4.
34. Lamb M, Jonathan B, Brooks E. How is virtue cultivated? Seven strategies for postgraduate character development. J Charact Educ. 2021;17:81–108.
35. Carey GB, Curlin FA, Yoon JD. Medical student opinions on character development in medical education: a national survey. BMC Res Notes. 2015;8:455.
36. Ryan RM, Deci EL. Self-determination theory and the facilitation of intrinsic motivation, social development, and well-being. Am Psychol. 2000;55(1):68–78.
37. Pellegrino ED. Toward a virtue-based normative ethics for the health professions. Kennedy Inst Ethics J. 1995;5:253–77.
38. Larkin GL, et al. Virtue in emergency medicine. Acad Emerg Med. 2009;16:51–5.
39. Weziak-Bialowolska D, Bialowolski P, Niemiec RM. Character strengths and health-related quality of life in a large international sample: a cross-sectional analysis. J Res Pers. 2023;103:104338.
40. Di Blasi Z, Harkness E, Ernst E, Georgiou A, Kleijnen J. Influence of context effects on health outcomes: a systematic review. Lancet. 2001;357:757–62.
41. Annas J. Intelligent virtue. New York: Oxford University Press; 2011.

42. Kristjánsson K. Aristotelian character education. New York: Routledge; 2015.
43. JCCV. Character education in universities. 2020. Available at: https://www.jubileecentre.ac.uk/character-education-/higher-education-framework/. Accessed: 1 Oct 2021.
44. Bruya B, Ardelt M. Wisdom can be taught: a proof-of-concept study for fostering wisdom in the classroom. Learn Instr. 2018b;58:106–14.
45. Bruya B, Ardelt M. Fostering wisdom in the classroom, part 1: a general theory of wisdom pedagogy. Teach Philos. 2018a;41(3):239–53.
46. Brant J, et al. Cultivating virtue in postgraduates: an empirical study of the Oxford Global Leadership Initiative. J Moral Educ. 2020;49(4):415–35.
47. Lamb M, et al. Commencing character: a case study of character development in college. J Moral Educ. 2022;51(2):238–60.
48. Glück J, Scherpf A. Intelligence and wisdom: age-related differences and nonlinear relationships. Psychol Aging. 2022; 37(5):649–666. https://doi.org/10.1037/pag0000692.
49. Aristotle. Nicomachean ethics. Trans. Crisp R. New York: Cambridge University Press; 2000.
50. McDowell J. Virtue and reason. The Monist. 1979;62(3):331–50.
51. Emmons RA, McCullough ME. Counting blessings versus burdens: an experimental investigation of gratitude and subjective well-being in daily life. J Pers Soc Psychol. 2003;84(2):377–89.
52. Grossmann I, Dorfman A, Oakes H, Santos HC, Vohs KD, Scholer AA. Training for wisdom: the distanced-self-reflection diary method. Psychol Sci. 2021;32(3):381–94.
53. Schwartz B, Sharpe K. Practical wisdom: the right way to do the right thing. New York: Penguin; 2010.
54. Cochran RF Jr. Lawyers and virtues: a review essay of Mary Ann Glendon's a nation under lawyers: how the crisis in the legal profession is transforming American Society and Anthony T. Kronman's the lost lawyer: failing ideals of the legal profession. Notre Dame L Rev. 1996;71:707.
55. Blasi A. Bridging moral cognition and moral action: a critical review of the literature. Psychol Bull. 1980;88(1):1–45.
56. Strauss C, et al. What is compassion and how can we measure it? A review of definitions and measures. Clin Psychol Rev. 2016;47:15–27.
57. Vachon DO. How doctors care: the science of compassionate and balanced caring in medicine. 1st ed. San Diego: Cognella; 2020.
58. Kaldjian LC. Practicing medicine and ethics: integrating wisdom, conscience, and goals of care. New York: Cambridge University Press; 2014.

Chapter 2
Phronesis as a Model for Surgical Education: Motorcycles, Bodies, and the Stochastic Arts

Margot Kelly-Hedrick and Ryan M. Antiel

Surgeons may be thought of as mere technicians, albeit technicians of very complex machines. This contrasts with what is perceived to be the more "cerebral" or "intellectual" specialties such as internal medicine or neurology. These physicians use scientific knowledge of the body and pathophysiology to hypothesize, test, and diagnose disease. The surgeon is then called upon for their technical skill. So, for example, a patient may present with a range of nonspecific symptoms: bone pains, weakness, fatigue, nausea, and abdominal pain. The internist does a careful exam, orders a battery of tests, and finds the patient has high calcium and parathyroid hormone levels consistent with hyperparathyroidism. They may order a bone mineral density scan and discover the patient has developed osteoporosis due to these changes. They order a neck ultrasound and a parathyroid scan and find that one of the parathyroids is enlarged. Since they have now made the diagnosis and localized the problem, they consult with a surgeon to simply remove the enlarged, hyperactive gland. This sort of teamwork and collaboration is necessary in medicine. There is no possible way that any one physician or any one specialty can possess enough knowledge to practice medicine alone. Surgeons must closely partner with their medicine colleagues. However, this example of a simplified clinical encounter can perpetuate the view for students and practitioners alike that medicine is about thinking, and surgery is about doing. This reductionist view fails to understand the types of knowledge necessary for good surgical practice.

In this chapter, we seek to situate the practice of surgery within the broader philosophical discussion comparing manual or technical workers to knowledge workers. To do so, we will engage the work of philosopher Matthew Crawford whose thinking has deeply influenced our own understanding of the practice of surgery. After pursuing graduate studies in political philosophy at the University of

M. Kelly-Hedrick · R. M. Antiel (✉)
Department of Surgery, Duke University School of Medicine, Durham, NC, USA
e-mail: Ryan.antiel@duke.edu

F. Jotterand, C. Bosco (eds.), *Fostering Humanism in Surgery*, New Paradigms in Healthcare, https://doi.org/10.1007/978-3-031-82771-6_2

Chicago, Crawford went to work for a think tank in Washington D.C. However, he quickly became disillusioned, having found the work to be ironically hostile to thinking. He spent his time drafting arguments for position papers that simply supported the interests of those funding the think tank. So after only five months, he left and opened up his own motorcycle repair shop in Richmond, Virginia. During this transition, he joined the Institute for Advanced Studies in Culture at the University of Virginia, where he wrote *Shop Class as Soulcraft: An Inquiry into the Value of Work*, an exploration of the nature of mechanical work, which he proposes is both technical and intellectual and requires a particular moral disposition [1].

In this chapter, we will draw on Crawford's argument to show parallels between the mechanic's work and the surgeon's work and explore how concepts in Crawford's exploration of "the education of a gearhead" also apply to the formation of surgeons. While we acknowledge that working on human bodies is not simply the same as working on a complex machine, both motorcycle mechanics and surgeons think in a way that is bound up in action, require instruction on how to direct their attention (i.e., they must learn how to see properly), and rely on tacit knowledge, which is related to the idea of practical wisdom (*phronesis*). These concepts have important implications for surgical education—residents require instruction from virtuous teachers in a particular moral community not simply textbooks or manuals. Finally, we turn our attention to the formation of *good* surgeons, which requires virtues not unlike those of a good mechanic. We touch on how the pursuit of surgery can inform the pursuit of a good life and human flourishing. In this chapter, we choose to focus specifically on how Crawford's concepts relate to surgery and surgical education, but we recognize that many of the arguments might apply to medicine more broadly.

2.1 Doing, Thinking, and Being

In the working world, thinking and doing jobs are often separated. Manual labor jobs—such as mechanics, plumbers, and carpenters—are often contrasted with thinking or knowledge jobs which do not involve manual labor but rather deal with abstraction and concepts. We have created a divide between "blue-collar work" and "white-collar work." The former work can be less respected in our society, often because of the perception that these jobs do not demand serious intellect [1]. We see these biases extended into the educational system as more shop classes are canceled with an ever-increasing emphasis on advanced placement courses and standardized tests in pursuit of matriculating at a four-year college rather than encouraging students to pursue trade schools [1].

Crawford argues that the perception that manual trades are devoid of thinking is grossly misguided. He ultimately left his work at the think tank to return to work as a motorcycle mechanic because he found it more fulfilling and meaningful. The bike shop was cognitively enriching and liberating—he "quickly realized there was more thinking going on in the bike shop than in my previous job at the think tank" [1, p. 27].

There has been a distinction between knowledge and practice for millennia. Broadly speaking, two main categories of knowledge from Greek philosophy are *episteme* and *techne* [2]. Episteme is often translated as knowledge or theory, whereas techne is translated as craft or art. In our day, pure mathematics would be an example of knowledge or theory, in contrast to structural engineering which is concerned with the practical application of mathematical theory (e.g., designing a bridge). Carpentry, landscaping, and motorcycle mechanics are other examples of techne. Yet, this contemporary distinction between knowledge and craft, theory and art, and thinking and doing is fallacious.

Crawford instead argues that workers in the manual trades engage in a type of deep thinking that is tied to the action of the work. Not only do mechanics engage in this intertwined doing and thinking, but Crawford also argues that there is a certain type of knowledge that only arises from doing that cannot be gained in other ways. One can read an entire motorcycle manual, but there is a certain knowledge that can only arise from actually working on a motorcycle [1]. For this reason, good mechanics have specialized knowledge and intuition that come from working with bikes for years.

The contemporary distinction between doing and thinking exists in the medical imagination as well. The narrative of a divide between medical and surgical specialties is likely rooted in part in the historical separation of surgeons and doctors. In Europe, surgeons were trained separately from medicine doctors in an apprenticeship model, outside of the university setting [3, 4]. Surgeons were, and in many cases are still, called "Mister" instead of "Doctor," excluded from medical professional societies, and viewed as part of the trades class, often practicing in the community rather than hospitals [3]. In the 1500s, surgeons joined barbers in their unions to bolster their credibility, and it was not until the late eighteenth century that surgeons split off from barbers and formed their own professional societies [3]. It wasn't until the early nineteenth century that surgeons joined medical doctors in a shared training program in the United Kingdom [3].

Today there remains a divide between medicine and surgery, in part due to a legitimate difference in method of practice and perhaps also as a remnant of the historical origin of surgery. This bifurcation is even present in our common language, for example, the "College of Physicians *and* Surgeons." Early in medical education, students are encouraged to broadly decide between medicine and surgery. It is often purported that the medicine specialties are the "thinking" ones and the surgical specialties are the "doing" ones. This narrative reinforces the idea that *doing* is somehow divorced from thinking, and thus surgeons just *do* and leave the thinking to the medicine doctors. However, this is far from reality.

First, the surgical sciences obviously involve episteme, and the expert surgeon must possess a broad knowledge of the pertinent anatomy, physiology, pathology, and pharmacology. Surgeon-scientists contribute to scientific discovery in both the basic science as well as the clinical and translational sciences. However, there is also a type of knowledge that only comes from *doing* surgery—a deep understanding of the spatial relationship between things, an appreciation for the strength and delicacy of structures, and a deep ability to improvise and problem-solve. This type of intertwined thinking and doing that Crawford refers to cannot result from just thinking about surgery or reading about it in a textbook. This type of knowledge and understanding can only be gleaned from being physically present in the operating room, working with one's hands, and even making mistakes and dealing with the consequences. But being present in the operating room is necessary, but not sufficient. This type of knowledge acquisition requires deliberate practice and learning under an experienced surgeon who can instruct the trainees how to direct their attention during the operation until it becomes second nature.

2.2 Learning to See

Crawford recounts the time he, after struggling to diagnose a broken bike, finally gets help from a more senior expert mechanic who immediately sees the flaw upon examining the motorcycle part. He writes:

> Countless times… a more experienced mechanic has pointed out something to me that was right in front of my face, but which I lacked the knowledge to see… the raw sensual data reaching my eye before and after are the same, but without the pertinent framework of meaning, the features in question are invisible. [1, p. 91]

Despite having examined the part closely himself, Crawford was unable to see the issue until he was taught how to look at the part. Despite existing in the same physical reality, Crawford needed a more experienced teacher to show him what to attend to in the situation and how to assign meaning to what he was seeing. When describing his shopmate, Thomas Van Auken, Crawford writes that he:

> …was repeatedly struck by his ability to see things that escaped me. I had the conceit of being an empiricist, but seeing things is not always a simple matter. Even on the relatively primitive vintage bikes that were our specialty, some diagnostic situations contain so many variables, and symptoms can be so under-determining of causes, that explicit analytical reasoning comes up short. What is required then is the kind of judgment that arises only from experience; hunches rather than rules. [1, pp. 26–27]

Surgical education requires a similar process of learning how to see and where to direct one's attention. Daniel Hall—a general surgeon at the University of Pittsburgh with training in moral philosophy and theology—likens this process to walking in the woods with a woodsman [5]. A woodsman walking in the forest with a city dweller will be able to point out how small clues like a tamped-down grass reveal the dwelling of a small animal or the presence of edible plants [5]. These clues are visible only to the trained eye. It is not unusual for the attending surgeon to be focused on one thing in the operating room, a junior resident to be focused on another, wrong thing, and the medical student to be completely lost as to what is going on, despite all three being present in the same physical reality. The attending can literally "see" what the trainees cannot. Hall gives the example of a cholecystectomy, a surgery to remove the gallbladder. To operate safely, the surgeon must identify and protect the main bile duct from the liver to the intestine. While a medical student or trainee can identify the pertinent structures on a schematic of a normal gallbladder neatly drawn and color-coded in an anatomy textbook, the anatomy in the setting of severe inflammation looks nothing like those drawings. The inflammation obscures the picture, and one can easily get lost and cause serious injury. Hall writes that he is "able to see the anatomy of the cystic duct even in the setting of severe inflammation because I have spent many hours in those woods, and if student surgeons will spend time with me traveling across the landscape of the human body, they will begin to see the anatomy for themselves" [5, p. 121]. Surgical education requires a process of learning what to attend to during each step of an operation, just as Crawford was taught how to attend to a motorcycle.

2.3 Tacit Knowledge and Phronesis

Through repetition and practice, a novice becomes an expert as they begin to see what they previously could not see, as they begin to feel what they previously could not feel, and as they navigate situations where they were once completely lost. As Crawford argues, this type of work often requires "hunches rather than rules" [1].

Both the motorcycle mechanic and the surgeon rely on tacit knowledge rather than just theoretical knowledge. Tacit knowledge is the "hunches." It recognizes that expertise draws on some level of intuition that comes from experience; it describes knowledge that is present but cannot be fully articulated [6]. Tacit knowledge "encompasses elements of techne and episteme that are both learned and performed without conscious thought" [6, p. e489]. The mechanic, according to Crawford, relies "on a tacit integration of sensual knowledge, by which he subconsciously refers what he sees to patterns built up in his mind through long experience" [1, p. 172].

Another example Crawford offers is that of experienced firefighters who rely on tacit knowledge to know when a building is about to collapse from a fire. Over time, having watched countless structures burn down, the seasoned firefighter can integrate perceptual information and build strong pattern recognition skills that result in the development of this "sixth sense," though they may not be able to state exactly how they know a building is about to collapse [1].

Surgery also hinges on tacit knowledge. An expert surgeon makes hundreds of decisions in each operation, based on both explicit and tacit knowledge. When tying a bleeding vessel in the operating room, if I tie it too tightly, I run the risk of tearing the vessel and creating even more bleeding. On the other hand, if I do not tie the vessel tight enough, it may come loose hours later resulting in delayed bleeding. I no longer think about how to tie vessels, I just know. It is hard to articulate to a student how much tension is needed in various settings; one has to feel the tension for themselves and even experience tearing vessels. I have acquired this knowledge because I have tied so many sutures before. This tacit knowledge is gained from years of repetition, pattern recognition, and developing intuition to make good judgments.

The type of experiential knowledge necessary for mechanics and surgeons alike is what Aristotle referred to as *phronesis* [2]. Phronesis is perhaps best translated as "practical wisdom," and encompasses the ability to identify the morally important features of a situation and act accordingly. Phronesis is developed over time by deliberate practice [2]. While tacit knowledge is applied unconsciously, phronesis requires good and correct judgments made intentionally. The surgeon must discern, with the patient and their family, how any particular intervention aims at the patient's goals and ultimate end.

Phronesis is the centerpiece of what it means to be a good surgeon. As D'Angelo and colleagues write, "phronetic knowledge is the knowledge a surgeon needs to simply exist as a virtuous surgeon: it is the ability to take the universal epistemic knowledge of the human body, combine it with the technical capacity to fix the body, and make decisions on how to do this across complex environments" [6, p. e489]. This understanding of phronesis emphasizes the need for conscious and thoughtful decision-making taking into account both generalized knowledge and the relevant morally features of the decision. It is the ability to choose the right action in a given situation and context [7]. "Practical know-how," Crawford writes, "is always tied to the experience of a particular person. It can't be downloaded; it can only be lived" [1, p. 162].

When pilots Chesley Burnett "Sully" Sullenberger and Jeffrey Skiles successfully landed US Airways flight 1549 on the Hudson River following complete engine failure, they were relying on phronesis. After takeoff from LaGuardia Airport, the plane collided with a flock of birds causing complete engine failure [8]. After considering turning back to LaGuardia Airport as instructed by air traffic control, or to a nearby New Jersey airfield, Captain Sully realized that the plane could not make it to those runways. Instead, he made the decision to land the plane on the Hudson River [8]. This deviation from emergency protocols was a calculated and intentional move by Captain Sully based on practical wisdom. No flight manual, protocol, or algorithm would have suggested this course of action.

The incredible story of Captain Sully and US Airways flight 1549 demonstrates the importance of phronesis, or practical wisdom, in a high-stakes situation when things do not go as planned. Making this decision required rapid integration of past knowledge and current context thinking about the moral consequences of different courses of action. Following an algorithm or decision-making aid is helpful in certain medical contexts; however, these tools cannot replace wise experts. As Crawford writes, "when things get really hairy, you want an experienced human being in control" [1, p. 168].

When an operation does not go as planned, an experienced surgeon must rely on both their explicit knowledge of the operation and handling complications, as well as their past experiences with similar cases. Hall argues that the experienced surgeon has the "ability to recognize that all available techniques for resolving the uncertainty have been exhausted, and what remains is to commit to one particular course of action, and deal with whatever happens" [5, p. 120]. It is phronesis that guides the experienced surgeon in how to proceed in these cases. This resolve to act well in the face of uncertainty is necessary given the nature of surgery, a stochastic art; human bodies are each unique and complicated, which bring uncertainty and the real possibility of failure.

2.4 Stochastic Arts and Failure

Both mechanics and surgery are examples of stochastic arts. That is, they work on objects, motorcycles, or bodies that they did not build themselves. This may seem obvious but has several important implications. When a motorcycle mechanic receives a bike in need of repair, the problem may not be readily apparent. The mechanic must examine the bike and understand how it was originally constructed, how it has worn down over time, and thus what has gone wrong. As Crawford notes, "fixing things, whether cars or human bodies, is very different from building things from scratch" [1, p. 81]. Building things from scratch gives the builder control and understanding of the object. In contrast, when dealing with objects that one did not construct, there remains a distance between the object and the one approaching it. Aristotle describes this type of art as "stochastic" [2].

Surgeons work with storied human bodies with unique anatomic variances and often nonspecific symptoms. A good surgeon knows the generalizable anatomy and pathophysiology from textbooks but must also understand the person in front of them and diagnose what is wrong. As Hall writes: "surgeons can conceive almost any maneuver theoretically, but in the end, we are constrained by the limits of what can be done with the particular human tissue in our hands. ...Surgeons are ultimately limited by the given reality of the human body and its contingencies" [5, p. 122]. The recognition of the parameters and limitations of each patient's body requires an attentiveness to that particular person and an "openness [that] is incompatible with self-absorption" just as fixing a motorcycle that one did not build requires attention to the reality of the situation [1, p. 82]. Surgery also requires a kind of anthropology—an understanding about human beings as embodied beings in relation with others and the external world. The mechanic and surgeon must get out of their own heads and attend to the object at hand.

Even masters of the stochastic arts will fail. Failure at some point is expected because the things (or bodies) one is working on are complicated. The stochastic arts include aspects that are unknowable, necessitating acting within the confines of incomplete information. Those who work in the stochastic arts are dealing with particulars, a particular motorcycle or a particular human body, not simply abstract objects. They can recognize patterns and how these particular objects deviate from their class. However, one cannot always know the various forces that have acted upon a particular object. Samuel Gorovitz and Alasdair MacIntyre identify these obscurities in their important essay, "Toward a theory of medical fallibility," in which they argue that errors are inevitable in medicine because of characteristics inherent to the practice of medicine [9]. As an example of this necessary fallibility, they use an example from environmental science:

> Hurricanes and salt marshes, for instance, interact continuously with a variety of uncontrollable environmental factors. No hurricane is quite like any other hurricane, no salt marsh quite like any other salt marsh. Certainly everything that occurs to and in a hurricane or a salt marsh is law-governed, but because we never know what historically specific interactions may impact such historically specific particulars- for example, because of melting icebergs, flocks of migrating birds, changes in the temperature of deep sea waters, and so on-we never know in advance which the relevant law-like generalizations will be (even if we know them all) and which the relevant boundary conditions are. [9, p. 16]

Because of these variables, even the best meteorologists will have the real possibility of error when trying to predict the exact pathway of a hurricane. "What is true of hurricanes and salt marshes is thus also true of animals and people," the authors write [9, p. 17]. Surgeons are limited in their ability to prognosticate, and eventually, all patients will die. The master surgeon simply has to accept the limitations of their craft. Since mechanics and surgeons work on objects they did not create and which are not fully knowable, these crafts require a certain disposition to the bike and to the patient.

2.5 The Good Surgeon

While a good surgeon needs to be technically competent, this is not the only sufficient condition for the formation of a good surgeon. The work of mechanics and surgery requires a certain disposition—certain virtues or character traits.

Crawford tells the story of repairing a 1983 motorcycle by fixing the clutch and restoring its ability to run properly. However, while repairing the clutch, he suspected there was a problem with the oil seal, which was not currently causing issues but could cause an issue in the future. To fix the oil seal, however, would require a significant investment of time and cost. He describes "the lust for thoroughness is at odds with the world of human concerns in which the bike is situated, where all that matters is that the bike works" [1, p. 123]. Just because he *could* spend a considerable amount more time and energy (resulting in significant cost to the owner) does not mean he *should*; he must consider the bike's owner. Crawford sums this up as the tension between "your fiduciary responsibility to the bike owner and your metaphysical responsibility to the bike itself" [1, p. 117]. This in part requires overcoming one's own self-absorption to avoid becoming so entangled in fixing the bike that one loses sight of the context. Instead, it requires an appreciation of the moral contours of the situation, as these will help define the right way forward. To do this requires both honesty and humility—two virtues Crawford believes are necessary to practice the stochastic arts well [1].

Surgeons must also be focused on their patient as a person and their goals and values, and not just focused on fixing a problem like aberrant anatomy or pathophysiology. There are many times that a surgeon will encounter a patient that she could operate on; however, it would not be prudent to do so as it would not be consistent with the patient's ultimate good. This is why prudence, along with honesty and humility, is necessary for surgery. A good surgeon must know when not to offer an operation. She must be honest with the patient about the likely outcomes, even if the surgery is technically possible. She must also be humble about the limitations of both the body and the craft.

2.6 To What Ends?: On Human Flourishing

Crawford derives a deep satisfaction from his work not just because he enjoys fixing motorcycles but because of the satisfaction in helping others experience something meaningful and right when they ride. He writes, "my job of making motorcycles run right is subservient to the higher good that is achieved when one of my customers leans hard through a corner in the Blue Ridge Parkway" [1, p. 196] This understanding of a "higher good" is derived from a community of riders and mechanics—a community of practice. Crawford says "the narrow mechanical things I concern myself with are inscribed within a larger circle of meaning; they are in service of an activity that *we* recognize as part of a life well lived" [1, p. 197]. In this way, Crawford's understanding of the good life is connected to his work as a motorcycle mechanic and his participation in a particular community. This understanding of the good life informs his work by directing the aim of the work.

Similarly, surgeons partner with patients and their families to pursue treatments aimed at good and right ends. Surgeons do not operate simply to fix deviant anatomy; they operate to help mend broken bodies and to restore their patients back to their communities and work. Again, the surgeons' decision on whether to offer a particular surgery to a particular patient should not only depend on the technical feasibility or prospect of financial gain but rather hinge on whether surgery would help the patient flourish—that is, to restore them to a more nuanced notion of health. A surgeon may have a different notion of the good life than their patient, yet working within our diverse settings, the surgeon can seek to understand what contributes to the patient's flourishing and if a particular operation can aid the patient toward that end. If removing a tumor is technically feasible but will not relieve pain or allow the dying patient to return home to their community or work, the surgeon should not recommend proceeding. Ultimately, the pursuit of the patient's flourishing should direct the work.

2.7 Implications for Surgical Education

In summary, a good surgeon must build tacit knowledge and phronesis from experience. This has significant implications for surgical education. How might Crawford's description of the formation of good motorcycle mechanics guide our understanding of the formation of good surgeons?

The first implication is that the formation of a surgeon cannot come solely from a textbook or the latest journal article, just as a motorcycle mechanic could not learn the trade by reading a bike's owner's manual. The manual cannot capture the discernment and judgment required to make good decisions while fixing a bike. The manual also fails to take into account the context of the decision-making. Crawford writes, "the factory service manuals tell you to be systematic in eliminating variables, but they never take into account the risks of working on old machines" [1, p. 26]. The manual cannot instruct a novice mechanic on how to take into account "physical circumstances that have no logical connection to the diagnostic problem at hand, but a strong pragmatic bearing on it" [1, p. 26]. Instead, this must be learned from those with experience.

Rather than rely on manuals, Crawford learned to be a good mechanic by working with experienced others. He introduces us to one of his primary teachers, Fred Cousins. When no one at the Honda dealerships could answer a question about a 1975 Honda CB360 motorcycle, Crawford was referred to Cousins, a motorcycle guru who works out of an unmarked garage on Goose Island in the Chicago River. Cousins taught Crawford how to see and think about problems in the shop—in other words, how to direct his attention to the things that matter. "Fred gave me a succinct dissertation on the peculiar metallurgy of these Honda starter motor bushings of the mid-seventies," Crawford writes. "He was a scholar" [1, p. 108]. Crawford goes on to spend several months at Fred's shop, learning as an apprentice. The work of the mechanic requires this sort of integration with those already engaged in the work. Crawford writes, "it would probably be impossible to do such work in isolation, without access to a collective historical memory; you have to be embedded in a community of mechanic-antiquarians" [1, p. 25]. He regularly consults a network of experts across the country who participate in an exchange of ideas and knowledge, which he dubs a moral community. The work of a good mechanic requires embedment in this moral community of practice, where individuals are tied together by a shared history, commitment to virtues necessary for the practice, and pursuit of the same end, which is the "good" of motorcycle riding [1].

The formation of surgeons, like mechanics, absolutely requires an apprenticeship under experts. The type of thinking and knowledge necessary for surgical practice arises from doing. The hands-on experience is how the young surgeon develops tacit knowledge. The integration of explicit and intuitive knowledge to make complex decisions is best learned by watching others do the same and, in turn, having experts watch and critique one's own actions. Hall describes this phenomenon:

> The conduct of an operation is not like following the owner's manual for a piece of furniture that arrives with "some assembly required." Even the most detailed description of the technical steps of an operation will not prepare the surgeon for the hundreds of small decisions that must be made: Where should I cut? How should I dissect this tissue plane? What instrument should I use? How hard can I push, pull or tear this particular piece of tissue? Where can I cut safely? Do I staple or do I sew? What can I get away with for the sake of expedience and what limits must I not cross? [5, p. 115]

As Hall notes, learning to make these hundreds of small decisions in each surgery can only be adequately learned under an expert, repeatedly being involved in the same surgeries over time [5].

Even after residency and fellowship, surgeons remain part of a moral community of practice. Attending surgeons frequently call on their colleagues for ideas, support, and feedback on cases. Morbidity and mortality conferences are a formalized way that this type of exchange happens [10]. This type of exchange provides a surgeon with accountability—the opportunity to assess her own technical skills and judgment, decision-making, as well as character, further feeding into her professional and moral development [5].

Training in an apprenticeship model and embedment in a community of practice is the basis of how we train the next generation of surgeons. However, it is important to be explicit in *why* we train surgeons this way so that as our training programs evolve and the landscape of healthcare changes; we can prioritize what is important in surgical education. Duty hour reforms have undergone fierce debate in recent years. We agree with efforts to reduce nonessential clerical work that can bog down trainees; however, there is no substitute for time in the operating room with an experienced teacher. As time becomes more restricted, we must prioritize residents' time in the operating room and wards with expert teachers. Through deliberate practice our trainees will habituate the techniques as well as character to become wise surgeons.

We are interested in producing not just technically competent surgeons but good surgeons. Crawford notes that this type of work involves a "mutual entanglement of intellectual qualities with moral qualities" [1, p. 73]. As of late, surgical education focuses primarily on the technical skills to practice surgery, which again is necessary but not sufficient for creating good surgeons [6]. Here, our conception of surgery suggests we ought to pay direct attention to the formation of a surgeon's character during their training (traits such as courage, humility, gratitude, composure, trustworthiness, compassion, honesty, justice, resiliency, and wisdom). Aristotle posited that character was formed through deliberative and repetitive practice, in the same way that one learns to tie knots [2]. With time these traits become habituated—a second nature. Surgical education ought to deliberately discuss character formation as one of its aims. Focusing solely on the technical potentially serves to perpetuate the belief that being a surgeon is limited to only the technical.

There are several examples of what it might look like to include character formation curriculum in a surgical residency training program. Lamb, Brant, and Brooks have proposed seven methods to promote character at the postgraduate level [11]. These strategies include "(1) habituation through practice, (2) reflection on personal experience, (3) engagement with virtuous exemplars, (4) dialogue that increases virtue literacy, (5) awareness of situational variables, (6) moral reminders, and (7) friendships of mutual accountability" [11, p. 115]. Several of these strategies echo what we have already discussed—habituation, reflection, virtuous exemplars, and awareness of situational variables. These approaches can help with educational efforts by grounding them in a pedagogical framework. At Duke, the otolaryngology-head and neck surgery (OHNS) residency program implemented a program called the Surgical Training and Education Promoting Professionalism (STEPP) program which focused on promoting six virtues: wisdom and knowledge, courage, humanity, justice, temperance, and transcendence [12]. They did so via mentorship, daily "reminders" about character, and training courses for both faculty and residents [12]. These efforts can serve to guide future similar efforts to teach character in surgical residency programs.

2.8 Conclusion

In this chapter, we draw parallels between the work of a surgeon and the work of a motorcycle mechanic. This work is inspired by and grounded in Crawford's conception of the nature of being a motorcycle mechanic [1]. Both surgeons and mechanics learn the craft through experience which gives rise to tacit knowledge and phronesis. This work cannot be done in isolation but rather requires embedment in a community of practice and training under expert teachers in an apprenticeship model of education. Communities of practice, as Crawford describes of his community of mechanics, can help reinforce ideals of the good life, or what we should be aiming for. Crawford also proposes that the practice of both motorcycle repair and medicine are stochastic arts, which necessitate fallibility at times, and demand a particular moral disposition—or character. Surgical education must attend to the moral formation and character development of trainees. We hope that in making explicit this model of the epistemology of surgery, it can serve to guide future efforts for surgical education reform. Surgical education should aim to form not just technically competent surgeons but good surgeons who act (and cut) wisely.

References

1. Crawford M. Shop class as soulcraft: an inquiry into the value of work. New York: Penguin Books; 2010.
2. Aristotle. The Nicomachean ethics. London: W. Heinemann. Rackham H., translator; 1926.
3. Aggarwal A. The evolving relationship between surgery and medicine. AMA J Ethics. 2010;12:119–23.
4. Camison L, Brooker JE, Naran S, et al. The history of surgical education in the United States: past, present, and future. Ann Surg Open. 2022;3:e148.
5. Hall DE. The guild of surgeons as a tradition of moral enquiry. J Med Philos. 2011;36:114–32.
6. D'Angelo JD, Cook DA, D'Angelo ALD. If Aristotle were a surgeon: phronetic knowledge in surgery. Ann Surg. 2023;277:e489.
7. D'Angelo JD, Cook DA, D'Angelo ALD. Scrubbing with Aristotle: cultivating surgical wisdom through inflection points. J Surg Educ. 2023;80:1751–4.
8. Pariès J. Lessons from the Hudson. In: Nemeth CP, Hollnagel E, editors. Resilience engineering in practice. Boca Raton: CRC Press; 2017. p. 9–27.
9. Gorovitz S, MacIntyre A. Toward a theory of medical fallibility. Hast Cent Rep. 1975;5:13–23.

10. Elledge R, Brennan PA, Mohamud A, Jones J. Phronesis and virtue ethics: the future of surgical training? Br J Oral Maxillofac Surg. 2020;58:125–8.
11. Lamb M, Brant J, Brooks E. How is virtue cultivated? Seven strategies for postgraduate character development. J Charact Educ. 2021;17(1):81–108.
12. Schulz K, Puscas L, Tucci D, Woodard C, Witsell D, Esclamado RM, Lee WT. Surgical training and education in promoting professionalism: a comparative assessment of virtue-based leadership development in otolaryngology-head and neck surgery residents. Med Educ Online. 2013;18:22440.

Chapter 3
The Education of Surgeons in the Humanities

David L. Larson

The education of a surgeon in the humanities must start with the definition of exactly what is meant by "the humanities." In its simplest form, the humanities concern themselves with human beings and their culture in analytic and critical methods of inquiry derived from an appreciation of human values and the unique ability of the human spirit to express itself. A further definition of the humanities would be exposure to classic literature by both medical and nonmedical authors, music, art, philosophy, religion, and other forms of human appreciation that lift one's spirits and expands one's mind beyond their present level of interest or employment.

The need for study of the humanities in medicine was identified over 20 years ago in this statement of an insightful second year medical student.

> I have been told that there are two pillars in medicine—science and humanism. As basic scientists build up the first pillar during the preclinical years and neglect the construction and maintenance of the second, students learn to treat patients as they might treat an experimental mouse. Idealistic notions of altruism, honesty, and integrity that attracted many to the calling of medicine are mentioned in the white coat ceremony, talked about by deans, and then actively discouraged through the acculturation process. This is where transformation must take place. [1]

This chapter explores the importance and benefits of educating surgeons in the humanities from early in their training. There are, of course, barriers to surgical education of residents in the humanities. Regardless, there are a variety of strategies by which this education may be accomplished, instituted, and monitored. Finally, we will look at what a humanity-driven surgical practice might look like.

D. L. Larson (✉)
Department of Plastic Surgery, Medical College of Wisconsin, Milwaukee, WI, USA
e-mail: dlarson@acgme.org

F. Jotterand, C. Bosco (eds.), *Fostering Humanism in Surgery*, New Paradigms in Healthcare, https://doi.org/10.1007/978-3-031-82771-6_3

3.1 A Shifting Focus in Liberal Arts Education

Starting with the 2007–2008 recession, universities nationwide faced the dilemma of less money for education, and the liberal arts disciplines were among the first targeted for cost-cutting measures. This included education in the classics, philosophy, history, and art. Once institutions of higher education recovered from the recession, the pandemic of 2020–2022 disrupted education worldwide, and this, obviously, included postgraduate education. Many university administrators adopted the argument that teaching liberal arts is a luxury. This mindset was previously decried by Martha Nussbaum in her 2010 book, *Not for Profit*, [2] in which she considers neglect of teaching the humanities as a "silent crisis," not unlike the global economic crisis at that time. Although she has no objection to good scientific and technical education, her concern is that other abilities "crucial to the health of a democracy" will be lost in the "competitive flurry." These humanities and arts-related abilities include critical thinking, an approach to systemic problems as a "citizen of the world," and the capacity to think sympathetically of the predicament of another person (e.g., a patient, peer, or care team member). An attitude that recognizes the value of the humanities offers the hope of sustaining decent institutions across our divided and disparate society.

A group of Christian humanists, many of whom teach in small liberal arts colleges, began to contemplate the value of the liberal-arts education that they had spent their careers providing. In a recently published book titled *The Liberating Arts: Why We Need Liberal Arts Education* [3], the editors present 25 essays (by professors, administrators, and students) in response to common critiques of liberal arts teaching: Do we need this sort of education? Is it a waste of time? The responses to these questions and the arguments in favor of liberal arts education include (a) an expansion of life that allows human beings to flourish in their occupation, (b) the cultivation of the habits of contemplation and reflection, thus allowing pursuit of the highest human activities, to see and live life to its fullest, (c) to enjoy friendships with others, and (d) to foster the health of their communities. In a summary of a review of this book [4] Jennifer Fry, PhD, Dean of the Honors College at the University of Tulsa, suggests that "the liberal arts provide an education that meets the highest aspirations of the human person and education aimed at human flourishing."

3.2 The Embrace of the Study of the Humanities in the Medical Community

The wellness initiatives of the Accreditation Council of Graduate Medical Education (ACGME) have been a requirement of all residencies and fellowships for the last decade [5]. A portion of the requirement reads: "The responsibility of the program, in partnership with the Sponsoring Institution, must include: policies and programs that encourage optimal resident and faculty member well-being." Considering this dictate, perhaps the well-being of both faculty and trainees might be further aided by study of the humanities that follows a simple curriculum. The renewed attention to the value of teaching the liberal arts, noted above by Fry [4], results in flourishing of the individual. "Flourishing" is a more robust and descriptive term than "well-being" because, in addition to the happiness of "well-being," "flourishing" includes notions of character and virtue. It implies a kind of all-encompassing state of well-being, not merely excelling in one particular area, but achieving balance across all aspects of life. Instituting the study of the humanities in medicine cannot just be an aid to the surgeon's sense of well-being but also allow the surgeon to flourish in all aspects of their life. The American Association of Medical Colleges (AAMC) is committed to supporting the integration of arts and humanities, stating that "arts and humanities are essential to the human experience and the benefits to medical education go far beyond joys and pleasures." To promulgate this commitment, the AAMC has produced a monograph, *The Fundamental Role of the Arts and Humanities in Medical Education*, which provides an in-depth review of the role arts and humanities play in educating a physician [6]. Numerous US medical schools, including Harvard, the Medical College of Wisconsin, Indiana University, Northwestern University, and the Schulich School of Medicine and Dentistry, London, Canada, have curricula that include the arts and humanities [7–10]. The value of including the arts and humanities in a complete medical education is advocated in the paper by David Jones [7] in which he identifies that this education not only teaches empathy and professionalism but other character competencies such as cultural sensitivity, ethics, and listening skills.

The Board of Directors of the American College of Emergency Physicians has established a Section of Medical Humanities to provide a forum in which its members with special interest in the fine arts, literature, humanities research, and the humanistic social sciences can develop a knowledge base, share information, receive, and give counsel, as well as serve as a resource to others interested in the application of these areas to emergency medicine [11]. The Association for Surgical Education has sponsored poster sessions with topics such as "Incorporating Humanities into the Surgical Curriculum." [12] Likewise, the *Journal of Surgical Education* has several papers addressing the topic, including "Art in Surgery: A Review of Art-Based Medical Humanities Curricula in Surgical Residency" [13]. The authors of this paper provide a systematic literature review of this topic, summarizing the findings using a narrative approach. Of the 13 articles that met inclusion criteria, 12 employed drawing or sculpture in surgical residency training, while one discussed art observation to foster mindfulness, team-building, and empathy. Eight articles used art as an evaluation tool, two for didactic and archival purposes, one employed participation in art analysis to improve empathy and physician well-being, and two others describe courses in which art production was treated as a foundational skill. The authors concluded that, sadly, the incorporation of visual arts training in surgical residency is rare.

Johns Hopkins University School of Medicine launched a program in 2015 to fund residents and fellows of all specialties to lead "transformative projects" aimed at developing skills "in the science of art and personomics" [14]. This latter term was coined with the intent of more fully connecting residents with their patients and, thereby, rediscovering what attracted them to medicine initially. It is hoped that this might combat burnout by providing meaning and purpose to their study beyond their required academic responsibilities. In one such initiative, a photojournalism project, two plastic and reconstructive surgery residents planned to follow 12 patients over 2 years, with the aim of placing the patient's reconstructive surgeries "in the context of their larger medical journey, their day-to-day lives, and their personal identities." The residents hoped to conduct interviews with the patient's surgeons with the desire of highlighting moments of hope, unforeseen challenges, and the transformative experience of reconstructive surgery. Although the idea was to ultimately share the photos and interviews in an online publication viewable by staff and the public, their efforts and project were thwarted by Institutional legal concerns regarding privacy and liability matters. Regardless, the awarding of this project speaks to one of the goals of introducing humanism into the surgical curriculum: so that trainees may better appreciate their patients.

The *Journal of the Surgical Humanities*, now in its fourth year, has become a tool by which its contributors can communicate their humanistic accomplishments by enriching, with their articles, both their lives within and beyond the operating room. This quarterly journal is intended to both sustain and encourage faculty, residents, and medical students to integrate the humanities into their daily surgical practice [15].

Based on these examples, it appears that although all levels of medical education (e.g., medical school, postgraduate training, and practicing physician) embrace the study of the humanities as an important concept in training a fully competent physician, this validation is less so in the surgical disciplines. Reasons for this are elaborated in this chapter, but first it seems appropriate to consider the benefits and barriers to teaching the humanities in a surgical residency. Once a decision is made to initiate this effort in a training program, there are numerous pathways this may be accomplished and monitored. The remainder of this chapter addresses these topics and suggests what the results of this humanistic education in a surgeon may be like.

3.3 A Shift in the View of Cultural Norms by Physicians in 2023

In the *New England Journal of Medicine*, Lisa Rosenbaum, MD [16], drew attention to the changes in how young physicians view their occupation more as a job than a calling. This attitude may have predated the pandemic but was, nevertheless, catalyzed by it. Though many baby boomer parents encouraged their millennial offspring to pursue their passion, the millennial medical school graduate faced unstable labor market that forced them to work and may have compromised that "passion."

This fact, combined with the subordination of educational missions to corporate entities, resulted in an attitude that "sacrificing" for their desired passion became far less appealing. The recognized "delayed financial gratification of medicine," when compared with their peers in other occupations, resulted in a sense of injustice that has persisted since the pandemic. All these factors have had the result of producing a cynicism that the medicine they practice lacks the "fulfillment" they expected. This cynicism may result in a lack of recognition of the patient's pain, less than appropriate treatment of marginalized populations, and a tendency to assume the worst about patients. The corporatization of medicine has only resulted in graduate medical education trainees considering themselves a "cog in the capitalist wheel," furthering a negative attitude about their chosen occupation.

Regardless of these facts, it is still the responsibility of the present education leadership to train the next generation to derive meaning in their occupation and to treat patients who want a well-trained and readily available physician when they, or their families, become ill. How do we restore treating medicine less as an occupation but more as a profession and a way of life that brings meaning and purpose to each patient interaction? One way to accomplish this is to identify that this doctor-patient interaction is more than a transaction – it as a covenant to provide medical treatment to another person. This might be viewed as a sacred covenant based on a patient's needs and the physician's empathy, compassion, knowledge, and skill set. As Dr. Rosenbaum notes, "Medicine may seem morally corrupt, particularly to a generation that is highly attuned to systemic failures. Our patients may suffer even more if we respond to institutional wrongs by relegating medicine to the margins of our lives."

The crisis in the culture of our medical education system may be addressed, in part, by the intentional and systematic exposure to the humanities early in surgical training.

3.4 The Importance of Educating Surgeons in the Humanities

The Accreditation Council for Graduate Medical Education (ACGME), the only US accrediting body of graduate medical education, identifies "professionalism and an adherence to ethical principles" as one of the six core competencies that must be integrated into any graduate medical education (GME) curriculum [5] and, thereby, taught and instilled in residents and fellows. In addition, professionalism must always be practiced by both faculty and trainees, as well as paramedical personnel. Of the six ACGME core competencies required in the education of all medical specialties and subspecialties (patient care, medical knowledge, interpersonal and communication skills, system-based practice, and practice-based learning and improvement), professionalism may be the most important, yet difficult to define. Residents, fellows, and physicians are expected (and required) to demonstrate this commitment with an adherence to ethical principles that include compassion, integrity, respect for others, and responsiveness to patient needs that supersedes self-interest. Professionalism is not taught in textbooks, but rather modeled by teachers and mentors at the bedside, in the clinic, and in the operating room.

Altruism and compassion are necessary elements in a professional relationship with patients and peers alike. A study of the humanities imparts an appreciation and understanding of the surgical patient who should be treated as a whole person rather than a diseased body part.

Another consideration is that the humanities serve as an outlet for individuals and may very well aid in reducing stress and, hopefully, lessen, or, at the least, positively impact the high rate of burnout, depression, job dissatisfaction, and even suicide that has become so common in our post-pandemic medical culture.

The study of both medical and nonmedical literature, philosophy, art, and history enhances critical thinking skills by inducing thoughtfulness and self-reflection, traits essential for effective and compassionate patient care that brings meaning and purpose to our training and beyond. With the rigorous and demanding work schedule during training and thereafter, a “less than caring” attitude, or even cynicism, may occur. Studying the humanities can provide an outlet to enhance selflessness and decrease such an attitude. Applied critical thinking skills result in better decision-making and a broader perspective derived from a deeper understanding of the ethical, cultural, and social dimensions of healthcare found in all surgical patients. These decisions will result in surgeons making more informed and thoughtful decisions in complex situations when they better understand a patient’s needs and their life values beyond the hospital.

Fostering a sense of lifelong learning may enrich personal growth. This will expand the surgeon’s worldview, develop a deeper appreciation for diversity, and cultivate a broader sense of cultural awareness, resulting in a more fulfilling and meaningful life both in and beyond the operating theater.

Another unexpected benefit of early education in studying the humanities is that it may provide an outlet for discussion and relation-building among, not just their surgical peers but all medical team members (e.g., nurses, physician assistants, paramedical personnel, and other medical disciplines). Meaningful interdisciplinary discussion that is based on something other than medicine may not only result in a trainee’s corporate growth but may also deepen otherwise superficial relationships.

3.5 The Benefits of a Surgical Education in the Humanities

The study of the humanities by residents may positively impact the entire model of surgical education; it may even be adopted by their faculty. This advancement of the humanities in medicine recognizes the complementary contributions of medicine and the humanities and further emphasizes the importance of engaging with the arts, culture, and similar leisure pursuits. As stated previously, an obvious benefit is to be able to recognize and acknowledge modeled professionalism that includes understanding, selflessness, compassion, and caring toward patients, as well as improving clinical communication with others and fostering observational skills. A more positive attitude and increased empathy are professional development tools that can be used in lifelong learning pursuits both in and beyond surgery.

Surgeons can cultivate and grow a sense of purpose and meaning by engaging with the arts and humanities. This will help them contend with burnout (e.g., insomnia, depression, anxiety, post-traumatic stress disorder, and other mental health challenges) while maintaining a sense of meaning and fulfillment in their careers and restoring the disconnect between health workers and the mission to serve that initially motivated them to enter a medical career. An appreciation of the humanities will nurture and develop positive qualities such as empathy, self-sufficiency, and efficient patient care.

The development of interpersonal skills within interdisciplinary teams, required of leaders in the management roles so necessary in medicine today, will further medical careers far beyond their training since these skill sets are rarely acknowledged in a surgery residency. Team activities will provide a chance to grow intellectually, personally, and corporately with others of similar interests, by providing focus on topics apart from medicine and surgery. Most surgeons are recognized as leaders by their community, place of worship, and business peers; early recognition and growth of leadership skills can only benefit a surgeon's impact on the sphere of influence in his personal, social, and spiritual life.

In summary, by early and intentional exposure to the arts and literature, there will be progressive growth in verbal communication and empathy skills that are critical for surgeons in developing strong relationships with patients and their families. When surgeons better understand and connect with patients at a more personal level, there is potential for a better health outcome that will always complement a successful surgical procedure or hospitalization.

3.6 Barriers to Surgical Education in the Humanities

After acknowledging the importance and benefits of surgical education in the humanities, it is crucial to recognize that there are barriers to this education. Most surgeons, and physicians in general, may perceive the medical humanities as an entity totally separate from surgery. There is a general lack of understanding of what the arts and humanities have to offer medicine. By necessity, the medical culture prioritizes scientific and technical knowledge over humanistic learning; regardless, it enhances the clinical application of that knowledge. Academic surgeons may view education in the humanities as a luxury, or even a distraction, from the primary goal of becoming proficient in surgical diagnosis and techniques. It is expected that there will be a need to educate the surgical community of medical educators regarding the advantages of having a familiarity with and knowledge of the humanities.

The culture within surgical training programs or medical institutions can also influence attitudes. If the training environment prioritizes technical skills over the humanities, surgeons may perceive exposure to the humanties as less valuable or relevant. Additionally, personal experiences and interests play a significant role. If surgeons have predominantly been exposed to, or encouraged in, only the technical and scientific pursuits throughout their education and training, they may be less inclined to value humanities exposure.

Like any other field, surgery is diverse, and individual preferences and attitudes can vary widely based on personal experiences, values, and perspectives.

Limited funding can also hinder any attempt to offer even the most modest of programs in the humanities. With a lack of resources, an educational institution may struggle to attract top faculty who can provide engaging and meaningful coursework in the humanities. Suggested solutions to this difficulty are addressed in this chapter's next section, but it is sufficient to say that thoughtfulness, innovation, and networking can overcome this hurdle. In fact, a surgical program that places even a modest emphasis on the humanities may attract "humanities-sensitive" faculty members.

In the education of any resident, there is limited time because surgical training is, by its nature, rigorous and all-consuming, with a heavy emphasis on clinical and scientific work. Incorporating humanities education into an already crowded curriculum can be a challenge. Many medical schools struggle to find the time and resources to devote to it, though many have established a humanities division in their university and/or medical school. Regardless, it might be introduced as an elective or in a grand round presentation, attended by all, once or twice a year.

The final and most difficult challenge is the resistance to change by all stakeholders when asked to alter the traditional model of surgical education. The introduction of the humanities in a surgical program must come from the leadership but is, by necessity, an organic process. Therefore, there must be a significant shift in mindset from those who resist this change because of their comfort with the status quo.

3.7 How Might Educating Surgeons in the Humanities Be Accomplished?

When the study of the humanities is not considered a "soft" skill, but one that is essential, a variety of approaches might be employed to institute the education of surgeons in the humanities. Any large university has humanities-based courses centered around poetry, prose, law, creative writing, philosophy, theology, historical studies, and ethics. Many freestanding schools of medicine frequently have a bioethics department that may be a resource of information regarding the humanities and its education.

Rather than isolated and elective modules of education, a more holistic and shared approach of the bioethical and medical-philosophical aspects might be considered. A brief presentation by a faculty member with an interest in the humanities about its altruistic value at the orientation of surgery residents and fellows could serve as an introduction to the humanities. Humanities education should emphasize small group and interdisciplinary teaching that encourages the use of creative projects to reflect on patients and themselves, both collectively and individually. There may be humanities courses already offered in a medical school that may be tailored to the interests of a surgeon.

An essential starting point is the appointment of a "humanities champion" in a surgery program; this core faculty member would be the "point person" on this topic and be versed in identifying, promoting, teaching, and modeling the advantages of education in the humanities. This "humanities champion" would generate a curriculum and identify a stratagem for its initiation. This education would be considered professional development (another ACGME requirement). It may be initiated in the onboarding of new residents and then reinforced at an occasional grand round presentation that might speak to the advantages and importance of this education.

There are many conferences and workshops available through the American College of Surgeons and the Association for Medical Humanities. Literature and art collections in medical libraries and museums related to medicine and the human experience are additional resources that may supplement traditional medical education and provide a richer and more nuanced understanding of patient care.

Mentors, physician role models, and programs that successfully integrate humanities education into their medical practice can be a valuable source for aspiring surgeons. A training program that emphasizes the humanities might be viewed by residency and fellowship candidates as unique and desirable. "Humanities-friendly" institutions and programs may provide guidance, support, and inspiration in one-on-one relationships and group settings. One such program at Johns Hopkins University aims to develop skills "in the science and art of Personomics," as discussed previously [14]. Another resource is the *Journal of Surgical Humanities* [15] that communicates humanistic accomplishments both within and beyond the operating room.

3.8 Monitoring the Outcome of Surgical Humanities Education

As with any new educational effort, there must be a method of monitoring effectiveness to improve quality on a longitudinal basis. The most obvious method is for each resident to chart their own progress through the curriculum by compiling a portfolio that includes assignments, such as a patient's illness narrative from their PGY 1 year or revising their personal statements in each successive year of training.

Small group participants may be involved in a long-term project in which they would regularly respond, using a journal format, to two or more questions, posed by themselves or an instructor that provide a personal perspective. Any evaluation must be a two-way exchange of information rather than simply data retrieval. The participants and their instructors are truly collaborators in their education in the humanities.

Surveys, or similar evaluative tools, of both the faculty educator and the residents, provide feedback, quality, and effectiveness integral to establishing benchmarks and best practices. Objective assessments, such as standardized tests, that quantify knowledge and skills gained by trainees and faculty should be considered a necessity. Examples used to evaluate outcomes might be a periodic assessment of communication and empathy skills, and critical thinking abilities. Patient feedback on the quality of care (e.g., empathy, listening skills, etc.) comparing those surgeons who have received humanities education versus those who have not might prove particularly revealing. Periodic surveys of humanities-trained graduates would also provide valuable feedback and, perhaps, testimonies of the appreciation of the humanities and its impact on all aspects of their career and life.

Finally, prospective studies that track the career trajectories of surgeons who have received humanities education compared with those outcomes of surgeons who have not might be another measure of outcomes. Other parameters may include identifying job satisfaction, burnout rates, and patient outcomes.

3.9 Successful Integration of a Humanities Education in the Clinic and Operating Room

An integration and appreciation of the humanities will be manifest in a variety of ways that may be subtle and nuanced but, nevertheless, important to all those with whom they interact. One of these is the ongoing practice of "active listening." This is intentionally incorporating active listening techniques that involve paying close attention to what patients are saying and then responding in a way that demonstrates understanding and empathy. This "active listening" produces surgeons who are better able to appreciate the needs and concerns of their patients and their families, thus developing a stronger rapport with them that adds meaning and purpose to the surgeon's role as a concerned and engaged provider.

Cultural competence is a critical component of providing high-quality patient care. Surgeons who are knowledgeable of cultural differences may better understand and respond to the needs of an increasingly diverse and needy patient population. This may include understanding how different cultures approach medical care, as well as how a patient's worldview, cultural history, religious beliefs, and values may impact a patient's health. This is particularly important in the ever more diverse culture we live in.

A humanities-educated surgeon may incorporate narrative medicine by using storytelling and other narrative techniques (e.g., sharing personal or family experiences) to share and develop a deeper understanding of a patient's experience, thereby gaining the patient's perspective of a proposed surgery and/or other adjunctive treatments.

Incorporating art and literature into the clinical setting can provide a valuable source of inspiration and insight for surgeons and their patients. This may involve displaying art in the clinic or reading literature related to medicine and the human experience, such as the classic surgical texts of Halstead, Osler, and Blaylock and spiritual reflections of Paul Brand, the world-renowned hand surgeon. There is also more recent fiction authored by physicians that might be considered, such as Dr. Abraham Verghese's *Cutting for Stone* or *The Covenant of Water*, both New York Times bestsellers.

3.10 The Result of Incorporating Study of the Humanities into a Surgical Curriculum

In conclusion, studying of the humanities from the first days of graduate medical education can result in its eventual incorporation into a surgical practice that will broaden and stretch the natural intellectual pursuits of a surgeon. Examples of these pursuits might include collaboration with humanities authorities, such as writers, artists, and philosophers, to develop a deeper understanding of the human experience and how it relates to medicine and life beyond practice (e.g., retirement). These collaborations might lead to innovative patient care approaches, meaningful mentoring of residents and young surgeons, and a more fulfilling and rewarding career for surgeons.

References

1. Kenyon C. Transforming the culture of medicine? AMSA Medical Education Action Committee. Online posting, 29 March 2003. http://www.amsa.org/meded/prof.cfm. Accessed 24 June 2003.
2. Nussbaum MC. Not for Profit. Princeton: Princeton University Press; 2010. p. 7–10.
3. Bilbro J, Wilson JH, Henreckson D. The liberating arts. Walden: Plough; 2023.
4. Frey J. The price of flourishing. Wall Street J, 19 Sept 2023, p. A15.
5. Accreditation Council for Graduate Medical Education Chicago. Common Core Requirements. 2024. https://wwwacgmeorg/newsroom/2018/6/update-on-common-program-requirements/. Accessed 30 Mar 2024.
6. American Association of Medical Colleges. Fundamental role of the arts and humanities in medical education monograph. 2024. https://www.aamc.org/about-us/mission-areas/medical-education/frahme. Accessed 30 Mar 2024.
7. Jones D. A complete medical education includes the arts and humanities. Virtual Mentor. 2014;16(8):636–41. https://doi.org/10.1001/virtualmentor.2014.16.8.msoc1-1408.
8. Petrou, L, Mittleman E, Osiburn O, Panahi M, et al. The role of humanities in the medical curriculum: medical students' perspectives. BMC Med Educ. 2021;21(1):179. https://doi.org/10.1186/s12909-021-02555-5. Accessed 30 Mar 2024.
9. Northwestern University Feinberg School of Medicine: Center for Bioethics and Medical Humanities: Feinberg School of Medicine. northwestern.edu

10. Indiana University. Medical humanities course. Medical humanities | Scholarly concentrations | MD program | IU School of Medicine.
11. Emergency Medicine Board of Directors. Section of Medical Humanities. About Us | Medical Humanities Section. acep.org
12. Association of Surgical Education. Incorporating Humanities into the Surgical Curriculum. The Association for Surgical Education.
13. Cohen S, Dai A, Katz J, Ganske I. Art in surgery: a review of art-based medical humanities curricula in surgical residency. J Surg Educ. 2023;80(3):393–406.
14. Depasquale S, Zwolak P. Finding meaning through Personomics. Hopkins Medicine, Winter 2023, p. 8.
15. Mendez I. Editorial. J Surg Humanit. Spring/Summer issue 2017, p. 3 JSH_Spring2017.pdf. usask.ca.
16. Rosenbaum L. On calling—from privileged professionals to cogs of capitalism? N Engl J Med. 2024;390:471.

Chapter 4
Ethical Principles in Surgery

Marie L. Fefferman, Megan K. Applewhite, and Peter Angelos

4.1 Introduction

Everyday decisions faced by surgeons are often highly complex and have a significant impact on the lives of patients and their loved ones. While some decisions are purely clinical, most involve a delicate balance between medical, social, and emotional factors. Despite the frequency with which important decisions are made, most surgical training does not formally prepare surgical residents to make ethical decisions. Because of this, surgeons are often left to navigate these decisions in real time, educating themselves through experience rather than through informed preparation. Shared decision-making is influenced by a variety of factors, including the surgeon's clinical expertise, patient preference and condition, and social factors, with individual surgeons placing differing emphasis on each approach depending on the situation at hand.

Although many different frameworks may be used to understand ethical dilemmas, this chapter focuses on Principlism in surgical ethics. Principlism uses four principles to approach ethical problems: respect for autonomy, beneficence, nonmaleficence, and justice. Here, we discuss three clinical cases to demonstrate the ethical principles involved in each case, how the four principles can be used to help providers make ethical decisions, and how the principles often conflict with one another. When principles conflict, care must be taken to identify the principle that will act as the preeminent guide. By demonstrating the use of Principlism in these cases, we hope to emphasize the complexity of each scenario and both the value and shortcomings of using an ethical framework to guide surgical decision-making. Principlism, despite its imperfections, can defend against physician paternalism,

M. L. Fefferman (✉) · M. K. Applewhite · P. Angelos
MacLean Center for Clinical Medical Ethics and Department of Surgery,
The University of Chicago, Chicago, IL, USA
e-mail: Marie.Fefferman@uchicagomedicine.org

F. Jotterand, C. Bosco (eds.), *Fostering Humanism in Surgery*, New Paradigms
in Healthcare, https://doi.org/10.1007/978-3-031-82771-6_4

and, if all four principles are considered, unchecked patient autonomy. It highlights essential values that should be considered before reaching a resolution for each clinical dilemma. However, as will be illustrated, focusing on ethical principles may help clarify conflicts but is rarely determinative in deciding how to prioritize the principles.

4.2 Principlism

Although philosophers have utilized ethical principles to argue for right actions for hundreds of years, the use of ethical principles as an aid in solving ethical dilemmas in medicine has a much more recent history. The four principles most widely used in medical ethics analysis were formally described in 1979 by Beauchamp and Childress in *Principles of Biomedical Ethics* [1]. This ethical approach integrates elements of deontological ethics and utilitarianism to form a structured framework centered on four core principles.

The first principle, respect for autonomy, dictates that patients have the right to make their own decisions, free of coercion or external influences [1]. Particularly in the United States, autonomy is highly respected [2]. However, autonomy must be balanced against the other ethical principles, and we will soon make clear the potential conflicts that may arise. It is important to note that the meaning and extent to which autonomy is incorporated into decision-making may vary based on patient or local culture. For some patients, respect for autonomy means they are exclusively consulted about decisions in their care, whereas for others, autonomy may mean that their family is integrated into conversations surrounding big decisions, rather than leaving it solely up to the individual alone.

The principle of beneficence requires that the surgeon makes clinical decisions that aim to benefit their patients and serve them in a manner that aligns with the patient's best interest [1]. One can envision the commonly encountered tension between beneficence and autonomy, which arises when the recommendations of the surgeon and what is likely the "standard of care" are not an acceptable treatments to the patient, who has divergent thoughts about what is in their best interest.

The principle of nonmaleficence is closely related to beneficence and asks that the surgeon do no harm. With every surgery, there are potential risks. The idea of engaging in an operation that will necessarily result in a certain amount of patient pain and suffering is that the benefits *outweigh* those harms and that there is a net gain in the well-being of the patient. By intimately understanding the optimal balance between beneficence and nonmaleficence, surgeons and patients proceed with surgery.

The last principle is justice, which describes the need for fairness and equality in the delivery of care and administration of resources. This principle is sometimes overlooked since justice can be difficult to ethically conceptualize when a surgeon is treating an individual patient, especially in a dire clinical situation. Despite this, justice is crucial to ethical decision-making and must be carefully considered in each clinical scenario. As will be seen from the case illustrations below, the four principles of biomedical ethics can often help clarify why some cases are ethically more challenging than others, and the principles in and of themselves cannot provide solutions.

4.3 Clinical Cases

4.3.1 Case 1: Kidney Transplantation

The patient is an African American, 55-year-old male with a history of type 2 diabetes and kidney failure. He undergoes hemodialysis via an arteriovenous fistula every Monday, Wednesday, and Friday and has been on the waitlist for a kidney transplant for five years. After years of waiting, the patient's healthy 20-year-old cousin decides to donate their kidney to him. The patient and his cousin are a biologically optimal match for kidney transplantation. Both successfully undergo all of the necessary preoperative screening, including psychological evaluation. Since a living donor kidney is available, the patient is removed from the deceased donor waitlist. The surgery day arrives, and the patient is thrilled to receive a new kidney. In the preoperative area, the cousin tells their nurse that they no longer want to donate their kidney.

4.3.2 Case 1: Discussion

Justice is a critical ethical issue in organ transplantation since it is a major example of allocating scarce resources. With the current system, there are not enough organs available for allocation to all the individuals who would benefit. Specifically in renal transplantation, the supply and demand mismatch is enormous: in 2021, there were 786,000 individuals in need of transplantation, and fewer than 25,000 of these individuals ultimately received an organ [3]. A kidney transplant is a life-changing procedure for all patients with renal failure, and for some, it is lifesaving. Given this reality and the limited supply of donors, there are substantial efforts to decide which patients should receive a kidney and on what timeline. Despite these efforts, the current approach is fraught with inequity. In particular, Black patients are much more likely to develop end-stage renal disease compared to White patients but have been consistently less likely to undergo kidney transplantation [4, 5]. This disparity is deep-rooted with multiple aspects contributing to the problem, including structural racism, clinician biases resulting in disparities in care, and racial segregation in urban neighborhoods that bring social determinants of health to the forefront. Even the way a patient's glomerular filtration rate has been calculated is steeped in a historical neglect of equitable care [5]. Racial disparities are heightened for living donor transplants with more than half of living donor transplants in the United States going to White recipients compared to 11% for Black recipients and 16% for Hispanic recipients [6].

With this context, our case emphasizes that issues of justice may be initially difficult to appreciate but underlie nearly every clinical scenario that surgeons face, particularly in transplant surgery. Although this case may appear to be primarily about issues of autonomy, beneficence, and nonmaleficence, issues of justice emerge between the lines. Would this patient have had a shorter wait time had they been a different race? Would this patient have end-stage renal disease if not for the structural racial inequities implicit in healthcare access and delivery? Did issues of mistrust with the medical community contribute to the cousin's last-minute decision? The issue of justice is pervasive and critically important to consider. Surgeons must work toward obtaining justice for their patients and strive to identify injustice even when it is not explicit.

In addition to the analysis of the justice issues, which include, but are not limited to the above discussion, this clinical scenario also prominently displays the role of the principle of autonomy in the surgical sphere. The patient's cousin presumably has decision-making capacity and therefore has the autonomy to make the decision not to donate their kidney at any time, regardless of previously communicated decisions. To ensure that donors are not being coerced throughout the process of organ donation, it ought to be regularly communicated that they are allowed to freely withdraw from donating at any point if they change their mind. This is important because donating a kidney is not without implicit harm. There are potential surgical risks in addition to the possibility of developing kidney failure in the future. While the surgeon knows it would be in their patient's best interest to proceed with transplantation, this case demonstrates how the principles of autonomy and nonmaleficence for the cousin may supersede the principle of beneficence for the patient. If the donor's autonomy is given priority over the recipient's best interests, living donor withdrawal must be permitted even if the recipient has been removed from the deceased donor list. However, the principles alone do not clearly show why respect for donor autonomy should hold sway over beneficence to the recipient. Rather, we must look to the overarching societal value of respecting autonomous choices to understand this priority. Although Principlism can help us sort out why the case is challenging, it cannot define the most important principle in every case. In the present illustration, it is clear that in order to avoid the potential harm that a recipient might suffer if removed from a deceased donor wait list before getting a living-donor kidney, many hospitals will keep their patients on the deceased donor list even if they identify a living donor. Unfortunately, this practice may lead to further injustice because there is institutional variability in whether or not patients are kept on both lists until the organ is transplanted.

Physicians and policymakers are actively working toward new ways to optimize the number of transplant recipients. Principlism may, at least to some extent, help surgeons understand these new systems and make sense of an ethically complicated environment.

4.3.3 *Case Resolution*

Although we must look beyond the four principles to reach a resolution, we believe that the cousin should be allowed to withdraw their consent to proceed with kidney donation, even moments before undergoing surgery, because of the primacy of respect for autonomous choice, which has priority over responsibilities to benefit our family members in contemporary American society. As is evident, all four principles are at play in this scenario: the cousin's autonomy must be respected, the surgeon should not harm the cousin in order to benefit the patient, and the inherently unjust transplant system must be acknowledged and improved. Principlism alone does not define which of these principles should be prioritized. Instead, it helps clarify the dispute, and when the overarching priority of respect for autonomous choice is accepted, Principlism provides surgeons with an ethical argument for making this difficult decision.

4.3.4 *Case 2: Cochlear Implantation*

The patient is a 24-year-old woman with a history of schizophrenia and bilateral congenital hearing loss who presented to clinic to be evaluated for cochlear implantation (CI). Given the patient's age, cochlear implants would offer environmental sound awareness but would not contribute to the patient's ability to speak or comprehend speech. The patient experiences auditory and visual hallucinations on a weekly basis. She has a history of self-harm, suicidal ideation, and aggression toward others. She intermittently takes psychiatric medications and sees a psychiatrist regularly. She uses sign language to communicate and lives with her father and brother who do not know sign language. The patient and her family are very interested in pursuing cochlear implantation and understand the risks and benefits of the procedure. Based on known potential side effects of the treatment, the care team is concerned that cochlear implantation may exacerbate the patient's auditory hallucinations and thus worsen the patient's aggressive behavior, potentially leading to the harm of others.

4.3.5 *Case 2: Discussion*

Once again, we can look to the ethical principles to clarify what tensions arise in this case. Central to the argument against the CI is the desire to avoid harming the patient, that is, nonmaleficence. The patient's care team is worried about performing a procedure that could produce more harm than good for both the patient and others. Although the patient wants the CI and respecting autonomy would argue in favor of providing it, we need more data to better assess whether the level of harm would warrant overriding the patient's wishes. By examining the current data on CI, we can better understand how to approach this scenario. There is a direct relationship between the degree of hearing impairment and the likelihood of developing psychotic symptoms, yet this association is often forgotten [7–9]. Patients with hearing impairment can experience "musical ear syndrome," characterized by musical auditory hallucinations, and approximately 22% of patients who undergo CI experience this phenomenon [10]. Based on these data, it is reasonable to be initially concerned that patients with a history of hallucinations may experience worsening of their psychotic symptoms after CI, particularly when the procedure provides sound awareness but does not contribute to comprehension. However, musical auditory hallucinations are different from the auditory hallucinations of psychosis, and there is no evidence to suggest that CI worsens psychotic symptoms. The data, though extremely limited, suggest that this is in fact not the case, and patients with a history of psychotic symptoms may greatly benefit from CI [8, 11–13]. Meanwhile, there is no strong evidence showing that CI worsens harmful psychotic symptoms. One case study describes a patient whose delusions and hallucinations diminished after CI [12]. Another reported that patients' psychiatric symptoms were stable [11] while a third case report described a patient with rapid improvement in their psychosis upon partial hearing restoration with CI [8]. Notably, in all of these cases, CI provided some degree of improvement in speech comprehension, which is not predicted to occur for our patient.

Given the minimal data to suggest harm to the patient, nonmaleficence becomes a less important principle to consider. With the lack of evidence suggesting that CI may be harmful and the small chance of benefit, we believe that surgeons should proceed with CI out of respect for the principles of beneficence and autonomy. This recommendation relies on the fact that there is insufficient evidence to suggest that CI in patients with psychosis causes harm. Therefore, the potential benefit and the desire to respect the patient's desires outweigh the unconfirmed, theoretical risk of harm. As long as the patient has decision-making capacity and has clearly been informed of the potential risks of the procedure, both the technical risks as they pertain to the operation itself and the long-term potential risk of worsening of hallucinations, it is their decision to make. Our patient has a history of aggression, and although it is not clear that this is necessarily related to the congenital hearing loss, the safety of the patient and others should be considered, and incorporating the support of the patient's psychiatrist as well as any family they wish to have involved in the process is essential. Thus, we can again prioritize respect for autonomy since the evidence to support harm to the patient is lacking.

Without question, there are also issues of justice that can be identified in this case as well. Through a justice lens, patients with disabilities and psychiatric disorders are underserved and understudied. In this scenario, the surgeon is at risk of treating patients with psychiatric disorders differentially, despite questionable evidence that it makes sense to do so. Unless there are clear data that CI can lead to negative outcomes, a patient, regardless of psychiatric comorbidities, should be allowed to undergo CI just like any other patient with hearing impairment.

4.3.6 *Case Resolution*

The surgeon should proceed with CI given the low level of evidence that the surgery would result in harm to the patient or others. Here, Principlism may help to guide the surgeon more than in the prior case: it is beneficent and just to respect the patient's autonomy and proceed with her decision to pursue surgery. Meanwhile, the risk of harm is low, and there are limited data to suggest there may instead be a benefit to CI in this circumstance. Without the framework of Principlism, decisions in healthcare may be susceptible to biases such as fear of legal consequences or paternalistic approaches. Principlism encourages a balanced approach, which can be reasoned through, where the ethical components of this case are weighed against each other in order to prioritize the well-being of the patient and her loved ones.

4.3.7 *Case 3: Leg Amputation*

The patient is a nonambulatory 87-year-old woman with a body mass index (BMI) of 14 and a history of moderate dementia, congestive heart failure, and peripheral arterial disease. The patient initially presented to clinic with dry gangrene of the left foot and was recommended to undergo an angiogram. After initially declining, the patient and her family eventually agreed to proceed with the angiogram after months of return visits and in-depth conversations with the care team. When ultimately completed, the angiogram revealed unreconstructable peripheral arterial disease, and in the absence of acute infection or rest pain, no intervention was recommended. Over time, the patient's vascular disease progressed, and the patient presented to the emergency department with critical limb ischemia. Vascular surgery was consulted and recommended a left below-the-knee leg amputation (BKA), which the patient adamantly refused. The patient clearly expressed this preference multiple times on different occasions to different care providers. She felt there were no issues with her leg, and she denied any pain. Although she was conversational, her dementia limited her orientation only to self, and as such, she was determined not to have decision-making capacity. The patient is very close to her brother, who is her surrogate decision maker. The brother would like to pursue a BKA to "do whatever we can to keep the patient alive."

The hospitalist team taking care of the patient recognizes that the only appropriate intervention for this clinical scenario is the BKA as offered by the vascular team; however, they are concerned that an amputation will inflict substantial pain and that the patient will likely have a difficult postoperative course, causing undue suffering. They are struggling with whether or not palliation would be a more compassionate choice for this patient. Additionally, they feel uncomfortable abiding by the brother's decision when the patient, although suffering from dementia, consistently expresses an opposing decision, one that she has expressed many times before.

4.3.8 Case 3: Discussion

Certainly, a BKA is a lifesaving operation in many patients who present with this clinical picture. Forgoing amputation puts the patient at risk of a disseminated infection that could be immediately life-threatening. However, in this patient, the immediate surgical risks and potential postoperative complications must also be considered, given how frail she is. Given the patient's age, dementia, heart disease, malnutrition, and other comorbidities, the life expectancy for this patient with and without amputation is worthy of consideration. It is unclear whether her limb ischemia or other medical diagnoses would be the primary cause of further health problems or discomfort in the future. It is unlikely that surgery would improve this patient's quality of life; however, it does have the potential to lengthen it. Because the patient is malnourished with a BMI of 14, postoperative healing may be challenging, predisposing the patient to infection, and potentially necessitating further intervention and creating considerable discomfort.

In this scenario, respect for the patient's autonomy directly conflicts with nonmaleficence. The surgical team's challenge here is to balance the autonomy of the surrogate decision-maker to employ substituted judgment with nonmaleficence. Their job is further complicated by the fact that the patient's expressed wishes, at least on some level, are not concordant with the surrogate's decision. Given the patient's current health and limited options for an improved quality of life, the surgical team should emphasize recommendations that reduce the potential for harm. This case adds complexity to the concept of autonomy since substituted judgment via a surrogate decision-maker is required. The patient does not have decisional capacity—she was able to communicate a choice; however, she could not understand the relevant information, could not appreciate the situation or its consequences, and was not able to manipulate the information rationally [14]. The patient's communication of her choice should be acknowledged, and the surrogate must be aware of this communication. Nonetheless, without capacity, the surrogate should make the final decision using substituted judgment. Detailed and thorough conversations should occur with the surrogate to ensure that the surrogate understands their role. The goal of substituted judgment should be explicitly defined and emphasized, clearly laying out the most likely scenario this patient will experience if they undergo surgery vs. if they do not undergo surgery [15]. Doing so will allow them to make the most informed decision on behalf of their loved one.

Identifying wishes previously communicated by the patient at a time when the patient had capacity may be helpful. Particularly for this patient, it is important that the surrogate decision-maker fully understands the patient's overall prognosis. When patients or families say, "do everything possible," this statement can be a signal that there needs to be further discussion about what "doing everything" means to them. It may reveal an underlying request or misunderstanding (i.e., do everything so the patient can walk again or do everything so the patient's memory can improve). It may be more of a statement of emotion than a medical decision and sometimes reflects gaps in the understanding of the patient's illness, prognosis, and current situation. When there are little to no options remaining, this statement usually indicates that the care team should go back to the beginning with their discussion of the clinical situation. It is only once the patient or family understands the illness and has prognostic awareness that options, risks, benefits, and preferences may be explored.

Every effort should be made to relieve the tension that is created when a patient without decisional capacity vocalizes a choice that is different from the one their surrogate selects. Additionally, the surgical team should reflect upon their sense of obligation to offer the amputation, even when it may not be the most beneficial course of action for the patient and seemingly not in line with the patient's wishes. Sometimes there is nothing that can be done to relieve this tension. However, clear communication with the patient and family from all involved care teams can make a big difference in the patient's trajectory and the surrogate's ultimate decision. An honest discussion about this patient's prognosis may help the surrogate to make a decision that is more closely aligned with the patient's expressed choice.

4.3.9 Case Resolution

In this scenario, Principlism highlights the critical tension between respect for autonomy and nonmaleficence. The physician and patient should participate in shared decision-making, which must be informed by medical expertise and the best available evidence. Surgeons possess a deeper understanding of the patient's potential post-operative course and complications, especially in a malnourished patient with dementia and other significant health issues. Because there may be significant harm done to the patient by pursuing surgery, the surgeon may choose to specifically recommend avoiding surgery as opposed to providing both options as if they are of equal benefit to the patient. Nonetheless, the option to pursue surgery should also be discussed. The resolution of this case hinges on ensuring that the surrogate decision-maker understands their role and grasps the potential quality of life implications with and without surgery. Once this understanding is confirmed, if the surrogate still chooses to proceed with surgery based on their belief that this choice aligns with the patient's wishes, that choice should be respected.

4.4 Conclusion

These clinical cases portray the ethical challenges that surgeons and surgical trainees face. As the cases illustrate, Principlism can provide a foundation upon which surgeons may think critically about their own clinical cases. The four principles delicately interact with each other and at times conflict without clear solutions. Surgical decision-making will never be simple, but these principles can provide a framework for thinking about the arguments on both sides. While Principlism provides a general framework for ethical decision-making, it does not prioritize one principle over another, leaving clinicians to use additional ethical and moral strategies to resolve conflicts that arise from competing principles. The lack of hierarchical guidance may lead to potential inconsistencies and has led many to seek additional reasons for choosing what is "best" for a patient. For example, one surgeon may prioritize autonomy as the preeminent principle while another may predominantly prioritize justice. In practice, surgeons often supplement Principlism with other ethical approaches, clinical evidence, surgeon preference, commonly accepted standards of care, and personal values to navigate and resolve complex ethical dilemmas.

Acknowledgments None.

Competing Interests The authors have no conflicts of interest to declare that are relevant to the content of this chapter.

References

1. Beauchamp TL, James F. Childress. Principles of biomedical ethics. New York: Oxford University Press; 2001.
2. Varelius J. The value of autonomy in medical ethics. Med Health Care Philos. 2006;9(3):377–88.
3. National Kidney Foundation [Internet]. 2023. Transplants for all: saving lives, one kidney at a time. Available from: https://www.kidney.org/newsletter/transplants-all-saving-lives-one-kidney-time#:~:text=In%202021%2C%20there%20were%20786%2C000,receive%20a%20life%2Dsaving%20transplant
4. Purnell TS, Luo X, Cooper LA, Massie AB, Kucirka LM, Henderson ML, et al. Association of race and ethnicity with live donor kidney transplantation in the United States from 1995 to 2014. JAMA. 2018;319(1):49–61.
5. Boulware LE, Purnell TS, Mohottige D. Systemic kidney transplant inequities for black individuals: examining the contribution of racialized kidney function estimating equations. JAMA Netw Open. 2021;4(1):e2034630.
6. Addressing disparities in kidney transplantation [Internet]. American Kidney Fund; Available from: https://www.kidneyfund.org/sites/default/files/media/documents/addressing-disparities-in-transplantation_1.pdf
7. Linszen MMJ, Brouwer RM, Heringa SM, Sommer IE. Increased risk of psychosis in patients with hearing impairment: review and meta-analyses. Neurosci Biobehav Rev. 2016;1(62):1–20.
8. Sommer IE, Roze CM, Linszen MMJ, Somers M, van Zanten GA. Hearing loss; the neglected risk factor for psychosis. Schizophr Res. 2014;158(1–3):266–7.
9. Shoham N, Lewis G, Hayes J, McManus S, Kiani R, Brugha T, et al. Psychotic symptoms and sensory impairment: findings from the 2014 adult psychiatric morbidity survey. Schizophr Res. 2020;215:357–64.
10. Low WK, Tham CA, D'Souza VD, Teng SW. Musical ear syndrome in adult cochlear implant patients. J Laryngol Otol. 2013;127(9):854–8.
11. Herisanu IT, Praetorius M, Mattern M. Cochlear implant in severe impaired psychiatric patients: a case series. Otol Neurotol. 2017;38(6):822–7.
12. Rebol J, Kravos M, Ložar M. Successful hearing improvement with direct acoustic stimulation in a patient with schizophrenia. J Laryngol Otol. 2018;132(10):946–8.

13. Filipo R, Bosco E, Mancini P, Ballantyne D. Cochlear implants in special cases: deafness in the presence of disabilities and/or associated problems. Acta Otolaryngol Suppl. 2004;552:74–80.
14. Appelbaum PS, Grisso T. Assessing patients' capacities to consent to treatment. N Engl J Med. 1988;319(25):1635–8.
15. Kruser JM, Nabozny MJ, Steffens NM, Brasel KJ, Campbell TC, Gaines ME, et al. "Best case/worst case": qualitative evaluation of a novel communication tool for difficult in-the-moment surgical decisions. J Am Geriatr Soc. 2015;63(9):1805–11.

Chapter 5
Why Do We Need a Qualitative Philosophy of Surgery?

Antti Huotarinen and Pia Sorto

5.1 Introduction

As the philosophy of surgery is specific and nuanced, it deviates from conservative medical specialties and cannot be effectively understood through general medical philosophy. Conservative medical fields such as medicine [1] and psychiatry [2] have started to define their philosophy. The subspecialties of surgery, specifically neurosurgery, have discussed a philosophy through the scope of metaphysics, epistemology, and value theory [3]. However, a comprehensive philosophy of surgery still awaits crystallization. *La Philosophie de la Chirurgie* by René Leriche from 1951 is one of the few books available. Despite being a nonphilosophical book, it touches on issues such as "thinking on surgery, its methods, and features required in those who serve." The book attempts to "define the spirit of surgery" [4]. Biographies are primarily utilized to discuss the personal philosophies of surgeons gained through performing surgery and their empirical knowledge of the profession. Examples of such memoirs and biographies can be seen in those of Carrel, Gawande, Marsh, and Sauerbruch [5–8] or in monograph textbooks. Sincere efforts are found in educational literature [9, 10]. The experience of surgeons remains alive through instrumentation, such as "Crawford," the incisions like "Kocher's," the procedures like "Cloward," and ways to operate, such as the concept of "Yasargil's microneurosurgery" [11], or the traumatological concept of "damage control surgery" [12].

Surgeons are perhaps rarely considered natural philosophers. The general audience, and maybe surgeons, are in the center of a Venn diagram consisting of a cool

A. Huotarinen (✉)
Department of Neurosurgery, Kuopio University Hospital and Institute of Clinical Medicine—Neurosurgery, University of Eastern Finland, Kuopio, Finland

P. Sorto
Department of Neurosurgery, Helsinki University Hospital, Helsinki, Finland
e-mail: Pia.sorto@helsinki.fi

F. Jotterand, C. Bosco (eds.), *Fostering Humanism in Surgery*, New Paradigms in Healthcare, https://doi.org/10.1007/978-3-031-82771-6_5

school bully, a cold scientist-engineer, and a skillful craftsman-McGyver. The heightened sensitivity toward the surrounding reality and a tendency to spontaneously develop a philosophy might go unnoticed. Surgeons often exchange very personal accounts of surgical understanding built through considerable surgery experience, and master-apprentice interaction is essential in teaching surgery. Surgeons experience both fearsome and beautiful events in their work, as the outcome of the patient depends on their personal judgment, skill, and actions. These repeated events might contribute to the perception that non-surgeons mystify surgery and surgeons.

We want to contribute to the emergence of a philosophy of surgery addressing putative ideas of how we find surgery to be different from the conservative medical fields. This difference is most clearly present in the direct interaction between the humans encountered in open surgery. The training for masterful performing of surgery, the requirement of temporarily shutting down empathy during the operation, and the ability to cope with failures due to lack of personal skill and judgment, as well as the sensual pleasure of the unique operative landscapes and the sometimes intoxicating state of flow while performing surgery together compose the experience of the operating surgeon.

5.1.1 A Surgeon Is Forged in the Experience

High-quality surgeons may not be easy to recognize [13]. Experience is a surgeon's most revered quality and is considered a major factor behind good surgical outcomes. Experience is often regarded as a quantitative measure, such as the number of operations performed. Such metrics presented by surgeons positively correlate with the outcome of many procedures [14]. The more experienced surgeon has a better understanding of nuanced cases compared to the inexperienced surgeon. For a less experienced surgeon, it could be reckless to proceed with surgery in a specific case. In contrast, a more experienced surgeon could undertake the same case with relatively little risk, especially if it's within the surgeon's subspecialty. High-quality surgeries are not based only on the number of performed procedures but also on intelligence, manual skills, and good teaching practices. The result is the correct movements performed in the correct order, using the correct force, in the correct sequence, and at the right time for the correct individual.

It is evident that surgical experience and skill also affect treatment decisions. Sadly, experience is mostly disregarded in the literature, and surgery is treated similarly to medical treatments where therapy delivery is constant and not dependent on the professionals' skills. Such sentiments cause tension between the importance of experience, understanding, and better judgment. The current emphasis on RCTs may overlook the value of a surgeon's experience when judging what cases to operate on and what not. Such disregard toward experienced and knowledgeable surgeons is consequently detrimental to the quality of surgery that is required.

A good teacher is essential to the development of a surgeon. Besides revealing the hidden moves in the OR, the teacher can transfer their thinking style, enhancing learning and the development of understanding. The surgical community regulates the balance between not operating in cases that are too difficult and staying out of the comfort zone. As Leriche described the different styles of surgeons, it should not be necessary to require all surgeons to follow the same path in their development as long as the quality of surgery remains high. However, sometimes it seems that certain personality types fit better for different types of surgeries, such as elective versus emergency patients.

5.1.2 The Philosophy of Surgery: An Analytical Approach to the World of Subjective Experiences

Is it possible to approach the experience of having surgical expertise from a more analytical viewpoint? As surgeons, we take pride in our ability to scrutinize our actions and clinical judgments. Surgeons frequently communicate their experiences using qualitative language, but in medicine, such qualitative methods are sometimes dismissed. This limits the communication and analysis of surgeons' personal experiences and leads to a narrower view of the surgical profession and its work. It is essential to recognize and describe the uniqueness of our daily struggles and experiential viewpoints and analyze these more systematically. There are several questions and interesting perspectives that can be drawn from the surgical universe and the surgeon's experience from different philosophical perspectives. If we neglect this approach, we are arguably doomed to somewhat naive forms of communication, at least in an academic philosophical sense, or to loneliness, neither of which benefits us surgeons, our surgical practice, or our patients. To overcome this, we would like to benefit from outside traditions to better communicate our experiences.

Therefore, it can be claimed that it is not only our privilege but also our duty to connect to more extensive traditions of academic inquiry, even though they may not be directly accessible to us. Approaching surgical experience through a more analytical viewpoint could help us better understand our field and communicate such knowledge academically. In a philosophical sense, the subject of surgery should not be attributed to analytical external thinking but rather to a close examination of the surgeon's own experiences. Here, we present a more in-person description of parts of our work and bring them under scrutiny by academic traditions examining the nature of subjective experience and understanding. To address these in a more formal academic style, we propose phenomenology, hermeneutics, and aesthetics as areas of philosophical inquiry of surgery. Our effort is not exhaustive in uncovering all approaches to surgical philosophy.

5.2 Applying Phenomenology on the Experience of the Surgeon

While operating on a patient, the surgeon is in a unique position that raises philosophical questions outside the scope of modern medical philosophy. As the cosmos of the surgical experience is not available to anyone other than the doctors of the operative specialties of medicine, modern medical philosophy cannot effectively address such topics. We suggest phenomenology at the genesis of this exploration as it necessitates including qualitative approaches and experiences through an academic framework.

Phenomenology is a branch of philosophy that studies the world as experienced by a subject, a subjectivity, or consciousness [15]. Phenomenology deals with personal life experiences, rendering a seemingly evident surgical application. The analytical medical philosophy, which juxtaposes a phenomenological approach, includes an outside or third-person view of circumstances and actions, analyzed as they are observed in the world out there as opposed to experience, which are more pronounced. This presumed outside view directly conflict with the first person experience of the surgeon during surgical operations. Accepting that delivering surgical therapies rely on surgeons' immediate perceptions and necessity of personal judgment challenges classical analytical philosophy as a core concept of describing surgery. Surgeons need to be more than analytical observers and algorithm machines. In order to describe, understand, and improve our core activities in the operation room, we need to embrace the messier and more personal nature of our business in a systematic manner.

A phenomenological approach to understanding should be naturally suitable for surgeons as it deals with how something appears to the observer instead of a third-person view of the qualities of the observed object [16]. This somewhat resembles the distinction of surgical anatomy, where the operative approach defines the viewpoint and the possibilities to explore the structure against textbook-style classical anatomy, where structures are analyzed free from the approach's constraints and even the patient's living body. It seems very straightforward and natural for a surgeon that mental states are always directed toward an object (intentionality) and that one has to engage bodily with the object and the world. Similarly, one has to directly experience the conduct of surgery when learning to understand surgery, which can only be done in the operating room. A philosophical articulation in defense of a surgeon's continuing and increasing presence in the operation room that is currently challenged by many other responsibilities would most likely be welcomed by most surgeons.

By exploring some phenomenological terms and relating them to professional surgical events, we can explore the potential usefulness of phenomenology, possibly uncovering important aspects of delivering surgery and being a surgeon, the secret knowledge currently only available for the "initiates."

A phenomenological approach to understanding should be naturally suitable for surgeons as phenomenology deals with how something appears to the observer as opposed to a third-person view of the qualities of the observed object. This somewhat resembles the distinction of surgical anatomy, where the operative approach defines the viewpoint point and the possibilities to explore the structure against textbook-style classical anatomy, where structures are analyzed free from the approach's constraints and even the patient's living body. Also, it looks pretty straightforward and natural for a surgeon that mental states are always directed toward an object (intentionality) and that one has to engage bodily with the object and the world. Similarly, one has to directly experience the conduct of surgery when learning to understand surgery, which can only be done in the operating room. A philosophical articulation in defense of a surgeon's continuing and increasing presence in the operation room that is currently challenged by many other responsibilities would most likely be welcomed by most surgeons.

By delving into some key phenomenological terms and their relevance to professional surgical events, we can uncover the potential power of phenomenology. This exploration could reveal crucial aspects of delivering surgery and being a surgeon, which is currently accessible only to the "initiates," underscoring the exclusivity and depth of surgical knowledge and the privilege of being part of this esteemed profession.

5.2.1 *Epoché*

Epoché is a fundamental concept in phenomenological analysis. It involves suspending one's theoretical judgment from the analysis of subjective experience. This prevents a theory-laden observation stained by assumptions, allowing one to appreciate all the facets of what is observed [17]. In simpler terms, it means approaching a phenomenon with an open mind, free from preconceived notions or biases. This priority of direct experience comes naturally and spontaneously to many surgeons. The ability to see as much as possible in the operating field and simultaneously concentrate on the substantive details increases with experience. Epoché should be active not only for the visual clues but also for the haptic clues, revealing the material quality of the observed tissue.

Observing before theorizing could describe some of the core requirements of surgical attitude toward perception during surgery, as it means the ability to see correctly. However, the surgeon cannot proceed with only an empty mind. While delivering surgery, one must remember the anatomical map and be prepared to see an unexpected structure and judge it correctly. Phenomenological epoché is spontaneously used during a sequential approach to a changing situation in the operative field, such as encountering unexpected bleeding, other intraoperative complications, or structures that may challenge anatomical orientation or interpretation of the pathology. In these situations, it is most likely the interplay between experiencing similar situations, including knowledge of anatomical variations and the capability to challenge one's previous mindsets swiftly. Success in these situations may depend on the surgeon's intuitive use of epoché or the capability to bracket out previous assumptions and surroundings outside the operative field. From personal experience (AH), sometimes, in these situations, the patient history or imaging results are better understood in a flash-like realization. Although surgeons probably learn to do this spontaneously, training to use epoché could strengthen a surgeon's capability to encounter the unexpected.

Surgeons have a significant role in the discussion of phenomenology. Their first-hand experiences, which can communicate the pure and naturally unfolding surgical journey, are as crucial as the more academic methods in enhancing knowledge transfer and improving learning and application to surgery. This emphasis on the value of their experiences makes the audience feel integral to the field of phenomenology, reinforcing their importance in the academic and practical aspects of surgery.

5.2.2 *The Folds of Flesh*

Apart from its mundane meaning, flesh in phenomenology describes the world's structure and functioning. Using Merleau-Ponty's (and Husserl's) concept of "folds of flesh," it may be possible to explain the development of a technician-surgeon into a physician-surgeon. The "folds of flesh" refer to the layers of meaning and understanding within the physical body [16]. This concept can contrast an overly direct surgeon who sees only dumb tissue to be operated on with a surgeon who understands the meaning of standard and pathological findings and tissue to patients' quality of life and humanity. Therefore, a more advanced surgeon can see within the folds of the flesh of the lived body, understanding the more profound implications of the surgical process. The "folds of flesh" concept is a crucial aspect of surgical phenomenology, as it emphasizes the need for surgeons to understand the more profound implications of their actions on the patient's body and life.

Additionally, an operated body, i.e., an opened body and a lived body, is a crucial aspect of surgical phenomenology. Modern surgical research often requires PROMs and PREMs (patient-reported outcome and experience measures). These measures can be understood as reflections of patients' lived bodies, which in turn are returned as a possibility to refine the understanding of the opened body and how the physical surgery folds back to the subjective life experience of the patient. In other words, these measures provide a way to understand the impact of surgery on a patient's life beyond the physical changes to their body. The "operated body" concept underscores the need for a holistic approach in surgical practice, considering the physical changes and the patient's experience and quality of life post-surgery, and it should make the audience feel empathetic and considerate toward the patient's experience.

The concept of an operated body can also be understood as an expression of the uniqueness of surgical touch, as touch is also studied in phenomenology. Surgical phenomenology is not merely a visual experience but a multifaceted bodily concept that incorporates a variety of senses. The idea that surgeons have eyes in their fingertips underscores that surgical touch is used for manipulating tissue, sensing tissue properties, and navigating the body, underlining the depth of the surgeon's skill set. In other words, the surgeon's ability to "feel" the tissues they are operating on is a crucial part of their skill set, and this sensitivity allows them to navigate the complexities of the human body during surgery, making the audience appreciate the intricacies of surgical practice.

5.3 Hermeneutics in Surgery

Like phenomenology, hermeneutics, an interpretation study, could be a surprising yet powerful ally in surgery. The very name of hermeneutics, derived from Hermes, the messenger of the gods in Greek mythology, resonates humorously with the role of surgical novices. Their task is often to deliver and explain the messages and answers of busy surgeons to other professionals, patients, and relatives. In the context of surgery, hermeneutics can be applied to interpret and communicate the complex and often subjective aspects of surgical practice, such as patient outcomes, ethical dilemmas, and the impact of surgical decisions on patients' lives. Hermeneutics can help surgeons and other medical professionals understand and interpret the various factors that influence surgical outcomes and communicate these effectively to patients and their families [18].

The study of interpretation and communication is closely related to subjective experience. Even without additional facets, surgeons can employ hermeneutical thinking when detailing situations where our thinking and actions depend on interpretations. Many factors influence interpretation, such as the surgeon's personality, history, culture, social structures, personal experiences, and language.

Good surgery relies on the correct interpretation in many situations, such as patient communication, teaching, and teamwork. More crucially, the surgery itself needs the proper interpretation of both the preoperative data, such as the patient complaints and symptoms, and the imaging studies, together composing a realistic view of the patient's condition, leading to an adequate treatment plan with knowledge of the correct timing, the goal, and the potential risks of the operation. An experienced and skillful surgeon has built an understanding of the relationship between the imaging data and the actual three-dimensional anatomical condition of the patient, being able to see from the images how it will be when operating the case. More often than not, the opinions of radiologists, conservative doctors, and surgeons differ regarding the images, and the final interpretation relies on the shoulders of the surgeon.

Interpretation of the subjective experience is even more immediate while performing surgery. Interpretation of the seen and the felt is necessary for guiding the optimal choice of tools and applied forces, such as during a spinal microdecompression in an area that has already been operated on, where it is crucial to separate a nerve from multiple layers of scar to prevent a nerve injury.

The scariest step for a junior surgeon is when the senior surgeon leaves the OR for the first time, and the young surgeon starts to operate alone, making their interpretations and acting upon them. The learning will be the steepest, but the mistakes are sometimes paid with the heavy price of complications, often laconically described as "part of the business." Following surgeries, watching videos, and reading educational material are necessary to learn surgery, but true learning happens only when the surgeon swims in cold water alone. Loneliness, eventually stemming from the personal responsibility when making the correct interpretations and decisions, is a significant stress factor for a surgeon. A dedicated tradition of studying interpretation is available for surgeons, and understanding surgical hermeneutics and its difficulties might ease this stress.

5.4 The Aesthetics of Surgery

Aesthetics is an epistemic approach to reality and what is beautiful, analogical with rational thinking or scientific inquiry [14]. Esthetic experiences are born through senses and imagination. The inquiry into aesthetics has linked beauty with divinity and absolute good throughout the millennia. More recently, the eighteenth century saw the secularization in aesthetics when the objective nature of beauty was questioned, and inquiry into taste and the subject experiencing beauty emerged—contemporary times linked aesthetics with other human fields, such as politics, and separated beauty from art, which remained a form of communication. Despite this, the pleasure intrinsic to aesthetic experience remains an unquestioned property of what is beautiful.

Maybe surprisingly, in the middle of the diseases, pus, tumors, and blood surgery contains beauty—esthetical experiences and the pleasure linked with them. Approaching surgery through the scope of aesthetics might widen the general image of surgeons and their humanity, enhance surgical communication, and allow the observation of esthetical phenomena to be considered as an approach comparable to hermeneutics, a tool to interpret surgical reality.

5.4.1 The Beauty of the Living Flesh

One of the first skills that the surgeon learns is seeing. This is practiced when assisting a more experienced surgeon. Seeing and touching the untouched, harmoniously intertwined, interesting, bright-colored tissues and cavities and pulsating arteries and veins brings the pleasure of intelligent realization and curiosity, as well as feelings of excitement and wonderment [19], features also linked to beauty. The surgeon will relearn the concept of the beautiful and ugly. The beauty of thc forms and colors is visual [19–22] and can be pleasurable in itself, an intrinsic quality of the object [19, 22, 24], and can be enjoyed without the cognitive capability to appreciate higher values [23, 24].

A surgical procedure aims to remove and fix the ugly and make the remaining as beautiful as possible. Paradoxically and excluding deeper analysis of plastic surgery, the escalation of surgical beauty is a situation where there is no difference from the normal. The biological machinery can express its original harmony and functional unity, which are qualities of beauty linked with the concept of health [25, 26]. The surgeon deals closely with fully living objects, the life itself, which is no less so in the other medical fields. Still, the crucial difference is the often way heavier, immediate consequences of personal mistakes potentially leading to severe and immediate damage—an aspect of the surgeon's work that is frequently overlooked by the other medical specialties, contributing to the loneliness of the profession and making the collegium of surgeons the only other people with whom to share these experiences.

5.4.2 *Surgical Decision-Making and the Beauty of Rationality*

The primitive subject enjoys the beauty of the sensory level but seeing enjoys the beauty of the sensory level. However, a more evolved subject can enjoy seeing the beauty of acts and deeds. Beauty is above mere visual beauty in movements, power, and presentation skills [21, 24]. While performing surgery, sensory experiences coexist with motion, guided by knowledge and experience. The beauty and the wisdom are fused. An esthetic surgery, for example, the removal of a tumor in the correct plane or the closure of a large and deep wound, is a result of a complex process, years of practice, and the proper interpretation of the haptic feedback from the operative field. Application of correct forces and angles and realistic approximation of one's skills are needed for a good result. According to Leriche, a good surgery is beautiful from the beginning to the end, the good surgeon being "… a person equipped with the pleasure of movement, attracted to risks, carrying a different type of soul" [4].

With experience, unnecessary movements decrease, and the operation becomes smoother with fewer mistakes. The naturally high concentration on cognitively high-value sensory experiences, immediate response from the environment, and the patient's life together increase the possibility of experiencing the beautiful state of flow, which is both pleasurable and efficient. The operation becomes smoother with fewer mistakes. The naturally high concentration on the cognitively high-value sensory experiences, immediate response from the environment, and the patient's life together increase the possibility of experiencing the beautiful state of flow, which is both pleasurable and addictive.

The beauty of rationality can be observed in reasonable surgery, such as a femoral amputation or the application of the Bogota bag: despite the result not fulfilling the standard idea of beauty, yet carrying the intellectual pleasure of a well-planned surgery, "beauty born of reason" [21]. Aesthetics in surgery has been considered, for example, in minimalistic aesthetics of neurosurgery, where a minimalistic approach is harmoniously bound together with rationality [11]. Minimum entropy has been suggested to be behind objective beauty in nature [27], but this could also be applied to surgery. Rationality in surgery needs both studying and experience to make correct decisions and perform the operations well.

5.4.3 *The Moral Beauty*

The craftsman can feel the satisfaction after the wound is beautifully closed. However, there is an even deeper level of beauty in surgery than in a successful operation alone. Ancient philosophers saw the Good as dressed in the veil of Beauty [21]. The surgical decision-making and performance escalate at the maximum achievable good for the patient, and we must rise to the good, as stated by Plotinus [21]. The most beautiful and effective surgeries are esthetical experiences with a living shape of moral truths, as happiness is the ultimate object of morality [28]. Performing the right surgery at the right time for the right patient is the most challenging part of the art of surgery [4].

In De Sublimitate, Longinus describes the truly beautiful and sublime as that which always pleases everyone. In human history, it is the wish for the other to be well and help the other in distress. This is achieved by surgeons who have high morals and are motivated to develop themselves as well as possible for the good of the patient. In decision-making, one should be as scientific and rational as possible but a good listener and sensitive to the patient's needs, striving for as good solutions for each individual as possible, performing the surgery well, and remembering their limits. Sometimes, in the name of the Good, the surgeon must make dramatic, even painful decisions, such as abstaining from operative treatment, leading to the death of the patient, and giving up the hopes of their salvation. Sometimes, good decisions hurt the surgeon's pride, such as letting a more experienced surgeon take care of the patient and giving up an exciting possibility to learn something new.

Moral skills are last to develop in humans [24], but in surgery, these skills are crucial from the beginning, and the path to learning them has sometimes required human sacrifices that will never be forgotten. "Every surgeon carries a cemetery with them," it has been said. Moral skills are last to develop in humans [24], but in surgery, these skills are crucial from the beginning, and the path to learning them sometimes needs human sacrifices that will never be forgotten. "Every surgeon carries a cemetery with them" has been said. Developing good moral sense eventually leads to developing good taste [29].

5.4.4 *The Master Is the Standard of Good Taste in Surgery*

As stated by both Hume and Kant [20, 22], some tastes are better than others, and the experienced one is sensitized with the most developed taste to be the best critique of specific skills [22]. To have good taste means the ability to make good choices (Blaise Pascal). A good master can significantly speed up the learning process of a surgery apprentice by sharing their understanding of what is beautiful and good in surgery, teaching the standard of good taste in surgery, and teaching the learnable skill of rational assessment of beauty, as formulated by Reid. Beauty can be shown to those who cannot observe it themselves, and they will also be able to understand and enjoy it.

The master can help the apprentice live with all the pain and fears of the profession, teach the unreal feelings when the irreversible has happened, encourage keeping up with integrity in the face of unfair treatment and understanding the causes of avoidable complications.

5.4.5 The Social Dimension of the Esthetical Experiences in Surgery

Beauty wants to be shared, and sharing beautiful experiences is an intensive form of communication [19]. The emotional aspect also enhances the formation of memories and learning, supporting the intellectual and scientific thinking of the surgeon. The light of beauty brightens the mind, the nature, and the matter [31]. Surgeons share the aesthetics and the pleasure of surgeries, which might be one factor, and this might be one of the factors contributing to the occult, the unreachable connection between the surgical collegium, making it harder for others to understand us. Learning to see beauty is the same as becoming more rational. The heavy price of the profession filled with heavy responsibilities and natural hardships is paid back in the multilevel esthetical pleasures of surgery, as nothing is as good as a satisfied patient visit at the postoperative clinic, making surgery an art that eventually communicates human feelings [30] and attitude toward each other.

5.5 Conclusions

A philosophy of surgery remains to be born. By continuing in the footsteps of the predecessors who have sketched the first steps of the philosophy of surgery, such as Dutta et al. [3], we have exemplified a few philosophical inquiries into the experience of the surgeon, which remains the most valuable asset of the surgeon and the most secret of its teachings. Starting this discourse could influence surgeons around the world to more openly discuss their experiences with others. Explaining the intricacies of surgery to peers and both peers and non-surgeons and discussing our experiences are essential to improving surgical education, technical quality measures, and technological interfaces. More importantly, it could give more space for a more extensive variety of communication styles and viewpoints, increase creativity and out-of-the-box thinking, improve learning from others, increase safety and efficacy, and eventually improve our surgeries.

Moreover, a mystical aura exists around the collegium of surgeons, setting us apart from the other medical doctors, leaving us vulnerable to external critique, potentially leading to damaging effects within the collegium as the standards for the surgeon's humanity remain unrealistic. We hope that by sharing the nature of our experience through philosophical discourse, we could offer our ideas to those who want to make further distinctions of the nature of surgical work and surgeons. This might help to reduce the stress of the profession by gaining outside support for our needs and explaining better our role in society.

To describe the core of our field, we strive for communication between surgeons and philosophers, suggesting an academic relationship. The study of surgery requires more than traditional analytic philosophy, medical philosophy, and bioethics. Here, we introduce phenomenology, hermeneutics, and aesthetics as possible starting points for qualitative approaches. As surgeons investigate academic philosophy and apply it to their experiences, it is possible to build connections between surgery and philosophy. Still, this effort to create a new philosophy of surgery should not replace classic approaches to the philosophy of medicine. Instead, it should supplement them, build upon them, and build upon them and, in some cases, gain authority to explain how build upon them, and in some cases, gain authority to explain how to apply the classic approaches better.

The scope and benefits of a philosophy of surgery, in contrast to a broader philosophy of medicine, have not yet been fully described. Still, we should appreciate both approaches where applicable.

The Aesthetics of surgery has been discussed by us more widely in a Book by Springer,"Humanism in Surgery" (2025, Eds. McFarland, Magalhaes, Mostwin, Genadry).

References

1. Solomon M, Simon JR, Kincaid H. The Routledge companion to philosophy of medicine. New York: Routledge; 2016.
2. Radden J. The philosophy of psychiatry: a companion. New York: Oxford University Press; 2004.
3. Dutta RR, Lopez A, Hsu FPK, Paff M. What is the philosophy of neurosurgery? Systematic review and defining the discipline. World Neurosurg. 2024;186:35–42.
4. Akça T, Aydın S. René Leriche and "Philosophy of Surgery" in the light of contemporary medical ethics. Ulus Cerrahi Derg. 2013;29(3):131–8. https://doi.org/10.5152/UCD.2013.2248.
5. Carrel A. Reflections on life. 2nd ed. New York: Hawthron Books Inc.; 1953.
6. Gawande A. Complications: a surgeon's notes on an imperfect science. New York: Picador; 2002.
7. Marsh H. Admissions: life as a brain surgeon. London: Weidenfeld & Nicolson; 2017.
8. Sauerbruch F. A surgeon's life. London: Deutsch; 1953.

9. Ibrahim EF. Activity theory and the surgical workspace. In: Nestel D, Dalrymple K, Paige JT, Aggarwal R, editors. Advancing surgical education. Singapore: Springer; 2019. p. 105–13.
10. McNaughton N, Snelgrove R. The role of power in surgical education: a Foucauldian perspective. In: Nestel D, Dalrymple K, Paige JT, Aggarwal R, editors. Advancing surgical education. Singapore: Springer; 2019. p. 115–22.
11. Okten AI. Minimalism in art, medical science and neurosurgery. Turk Neurosurg. 2018;28(2):307–12. https://doi.org/10.5137/1019-5149.JTN.18855-16.1.
12. Hirshberg A, Mattox KL. Top knife: the art and craft of trauma surgery. Shrewsbury: TFM Publishing Ltd; 2004.
13. Birkmeyer JD. Understanding surgeon performance and improving patient outcomes. J Clin Oncol. 2004;22(14):2765–6. https://doi.org/10.1200/JCO.2004.02.044.
14. Morche J, Mathes T, Pieper D. Relationship between surgeon volume and outcomes: a systematic review of systematic reviews. Syst Rev. 2016;5(1):204. https://doi.org/10.1186/s13643-016-0376-4.
15. Moran D. Introduction to phenomenology. London: Routledge; 2000.
16. Merleau-Ponty M. The world of perception. London: Routledge; 2004.
17. Morand D. Husserl's discovery of reduction and transcendental phenomenology. In: Moran D, editor. Introduction to phenomenology. London: Routledge; 2000. p. 124–63.
18. Forster M, Gjesdal K. The Cambridge companion to hermeneutics. Cambridge: Cambridge University Press; 2019.
19. Sartwell C. Beauty [Internet]. The Stanford Encyclopedia of Philosophy; 2012 Sept [cited in Sep 2024]. Available from: https://plato.stanford.edu/entries/beauty/
20. Reiners I, Seppä A, Vuorinen J. Estetiikan klassikot I—Platonista Tolstoihin. Helsinki: Gaudeamus; 2009.
21. Plotinus. The six enneads, on beauty. London: Medici Society; 1917.
22. Hume D. Of the Standard of taste. In: Essays M, editor. Political, and literary. Indianapolis: Liberty Press; 1875. p. 226–49.
23. Baumgarten A. Reflections on poetry: Meditationes philosophicae de nonnullis ad poema pertinentibus. Berkeley: UC Press; 1954.
24. Reid T. Essays on the intellectual powers of man. Cambridge: MIT/Cambridge University Press; 1785.
25. Diogenes L. Pythagoras. In: Diogenes L, editor. The life and teaching of significant philosophers book VIII. London: W. Heinemann; 1925. p. 1–50.
26. Aristotle. On the parts of animals I–IV. New York: Oxford University Press; 2001.
27. Deutsch D, Sainani KL. Q&A: David Deutsch. Objective beauty. Nature. 2015;526(7572):S16. https://doi.org/10.1038/526S16a.
28. Guyer P. 18th century German aesthetics. [Internet]. Stanford Encyclopedia of Philosophy; 2007 January. [cited in Sept 2024]. Available from: Plato.stanford.edu/entries/aesthetics-18th-german/
29. McAteer J. The thirds earl of shaftesbury. [Internet] Internet Encyclopedia of Philosophy; [cited in Sept 2024]. Available from: iep.utm.edu/shaftes
30. Tolstoy L. What is art. New York: Funk & Wagnalls Company; 1904.
31. Ficino M. On the nature of love. London: Shepheard-Walwyn Ltd; 2016.

Part II
Practical Issues

Chapter 6
The Art of Surgery

Priya A. Rajdev and Nathaniel J. Soper

> My grandmother made a surgeon out of me. Born and raised on the reservation, she is a member of the Turtle Mountain Band of Chippewa, an artist, a teacher, our matriarch, and my first attending. She taught me Ojibwe beadwork, putting a memory into my hands that found their homecoming in the operating room. I spent a summer in her beading group, learning everything I could from the elders drawn together, but most of all from my grandma standing over my shoulder, coaching every move, one bead at a time, patiently letting me struggle and interrupting with words of wisdom at the opportune moment I needed to progress from helpless to autonomous. Hours passed like minutes. I had to be reminded to stop and eat, step outside, go to bed. I never imagined I would be a surgeon. But then, during my last clerkship of third year, a beloved format of teaching I had forgotten befell me: the determination to restore order out of chaos, to repeat patterns until the parts were whole again, to absorb teachings handed down through generations, holding instruments in my hands, sewing, the quiet, the focus, the hours that passed like minutes—it was magnificently familiar, and I was hooked. I was home. (Jennifer Erdrich, MD FACS, (Personal Interview, 2024 Aug 14) University of Arizona College of Medicine, Tucson)

The art of surgery is a phrase that carries implications simultaneously grand and mundane. In many ways, surgery is a job—one that requires training and study, testing and evaluation, service and transaction, a plan of action, and a tangible outcome. But no surgeon would define what they do in such discrete, dry terms. When planning a vascular anastomosis, some would focus on technical precision, others the aesthetic beauty of the reconstruction, and still others the gratifying feel of a perfectly weighted Castro handling delicate tissues and fine suture. When caring for a critically ill patient, some are inspired by the speed and decisiveness of surgical decision-making, others may appreciate the intricacies of resuscitation, and still others may focus on the opportunity to develop meaningful relationships with the

P. A. Rajdev (✉) · N. J. Soper
Department of Surgery, University of Arizona College of Medicine, Phoenix, AZ, USA
e-mail: prajdev@arizona.edu

F. Jotterand, C. Bosco (eds.), *Fostering Humanism in Surgery*, New Paradigms in Healthcare, https://doi.org/10.1007/978-3-031-82771-6_6

patient's family. Therefore, we define surgery as everything that encompasses the practice of our field from the operating room to the patient's bedside, to clinic, to training, and to our day-to-day interactions with our colleagues and co-workers. On the other hand, the artistic essence that weaves all these elements together is more challenging to define.

In 2009, the writer and educator Mike Rose spent several months embedded in the Department of General Surgery at the University of California, Los Angeles. Rose, who wrote extensively on the value of trade labor and the relationship between mind and body in physically active jobs, wanted to understand the work that "involves manual skill but is high in status." He found that surgery fit this bill perfectly.

Sitting with then-Chief of Surgery, Ronald Tompkins, and a first-year resident, Rose asks the expert and the novice to review and discuss recorded footage of a laparoscopic cholecystectomy. Each surgeon narrates the operation with attention to slightly different details but with a similar eye on technique and tissue handling. Each of them describes how the cystic duct and artery are revealed with a gentle spread in the overlying fibrofatty tissue. Rose observes that even though the surgeons are on opposite ends of the spectrum of expertise, both express a deep appreciation for how the operation is a performance—an intricate dance between dynamic technique and the constancy of anatomy.

At one point, Dr. Tompkins tells Rose that laparoscopic surgery is like "trying to eat spaghetti with chopsticks—and doing it by looking in a mirror over your head!" Later, the resident describes the process of retraining one's hand-eye coordination in a very technical way, with equal attention to every small detail, betraying his perspective as a novice apprentice who cannot yet prioritize incoming data. But at the end of his explanation, the resident reveals a deep truth, telling Rose that with enough training, "you develop an eye for what looks good and what doesn't."

Reflecting on his time with the residents and attending surgeons at UCLA, Rose finds that there is something more to the art of surgery than "book learning" plus "technical expertise." In a passage that will feel familiar to many, Dr. Tompkins recounts that junior surgeons call him for advice about unusual cases or pathology they have never encountered before. He tells them, "Well I've seen it a couple of times, and this is what I did, and it worked out all right." Tompkins is careful to emphasize that a key component of a surgeon's confidence should be the understanding of their own limitations. Rose therefore concludes:

> There is a powerful tendency in Twentieth Century intellectual life to create mathematical or logical models to represent reasoning and decision-making. I think it would be pretty difficult to model surgical judgement. Surgical judgement is simultaneously technical and deliberative, and that mix is the source of its power. [1]

What are the granular components of surgery that give it this "power?" As surgeons, we have an insider's perspective that Rose did not. Every surgeon, whether in practice for decades or for days, has a notion of what we mean when we think about "the art of surgery." It's guaranteed that this picture differs for each of us, but perhaps we each carry an impressionist composition made up of all the same colors: technical expertise, manual dexterity and precision, deep understanding of tissue, innovation, adaptation, esthetic judgment, communication skills, empathy, collaboration, leadership dedication to lifelong learning, respect for tradition, an ability to draw from expertise in other arts such as music, painting, drafting, acting, writing, etc.

In philosophical terms, this grappling with consciousness of doing or experiencing a thing is called "qualia," or "the way things seem to us." Put another way, we will attempt to examine the "tacit knowledge" to which the philosopher Michael Polanyi refers in his explorations of skills that are only apparent because of the results those skills produce [2, 3]. In this chapter, we will grapple with this intangibility of the Art of Surgery, exploring the liminal spaces between the definable and indefinable, diving into many of these key concepts that all students of surgery will recognize in their mentors, their peers, and themselves.

We have found it helpful to divide our approach into two main sections: Surgery as Craft and Surgery as Art. Within the first section, we will explore the philosophy of craft work as artistic expression and offer a historical perspective on how our field evolved from humble origins as a trade into a bona fide pillar of the medical arts. In the second section, we will explore the so-called soft skills that are required to apply technical expertise to the right patient at the right time, and how an evolving balancing act between self-sacrifice and self-preservation may shape the future of our field.

6.1 Surgery as Craft

6.1.1 Philosophy of Craft

> Craftsmanship must reckon with the infallible judgement of reality, where one's failures or shortcomings cannot be interpreted away. (Matthew Crawford in *Shop Class as Soulcraft*)

We all have heard a venerated surgeon quip, "I'm just a plumber." Indeed, the skilled mastery of the craftsperson—the plumber, the electrician, the cabinetmaker—is a fitting correlate for the work of a surgeon: at its highest level, craft is equal to artistic expression. Like any craft, surgery requires practice, time, patience, observation, experience, and respect for the materials. In our case, the "materials" are precious, fragile, and irreplicable. The timeless appeal of working with one's hands is rooted in a deep-seated drive to create, mend, illuminate, and heal, to lend something concrete to the world. The immediacy of craftsmanship is a driving force as well—to perceive of one's work in the real world. In her 2015 address to the American College of Surgeons (Olga Jonasson Lecture), Dr. Barbara Bass echoed this sentiment:

> Our results, for the most part, show. We lose blood, our operations take variable amounts of time, our patients hurt and sometimes have complications, some preventable, some not. But nonetheless, our results, good and bad, do show. [4]

If the consequences of failure or even partial success are so dire, what catalyzes us to practice the craft of surgery? Working with one's hands—drawing, knitting, or playing an instrument—is certainly intellectually stimulating, with some researchers even suggesting that it helps prevent mental decay by engaging more areas of the brain. But why proceed with our craft when the stakes are so high?

In *Shop Class as Soulcraft*, a profound reflection on the value of skilled manual labor, Matthew Crawford discusses his experience as an electrician's helper when he was just 14. At that impressionable age, the immediacy of the work was deeply impactful: though the work was mentally challenging and physically arduous, he knew that at the end of it all, he could flip a switch and illuminate an entire room. In doing so, he proved his own agency to his young mind. His small but tangible contribution demonstrated both his competence and his value [5].

Similar "lightbulb" moments occur in operating rooms every day: the reduction of a hernia, reperfusion after endarterectomy, and a newly transplanted kidney producing urine before the surgeon even has time to sew the ureter in—the hands and mind working in synchrony, generating tangible, immediate, undeniable results. These moments are what draw us to this high-stakes craft and calls us to spend our careers in pursuit of mastery.

These moments are discernable as the outcome of "flow." In the late 1980s, the psychologist Mihaly Csikszentmihalyi proposed the concept of flow as an "optimal experience" that is the result of "the process of total involvement with life." Similar concepts of mindfulness and total presence in the moment have existed in Eastern philosophies for millennia, but Csikszentmihalyi proposed practical applications to help modern audiences craving the flow state. His research suggests eight key characteristics of flow: (1) complete concentration on the task, (2) clarity of goals/rewards and immediate feedback, (3) time dilation, (4) an intrinsically rewarding experience, (5) effortlessness, (6) balance between challenge and skills, (7) actions and awareness merge and the self ceases to exist, and (8) feeling of total control. Together, these eight characteristics neatly define a good day in the operating room [6, 7].

For expert and novice alike, the desire to continually experience this flow state, to enter into it and tangibly produce good in the world, is deeply satisfying and perpetually motivating. A novice craftsperson who follows in the footsteps of a master of the craft will stand in awe when observing where the hands of that master have been. Crawford writes:

> I was sometimes quieted at the sight of a gang of conduit entering a large panel in a commercial setting, bent into nestled, flowing curves, with varying offsets, that somehow all terminated in the same plane. This was a skill so far beyond my abilities that I felt I was in the presence of some genius…craftsmanship might be defined simply as the desire to do something well, for its own sake. [5]

Uncovering the inner workings of an electrical panel evokes the image of a surgeon standing over a widely open abdomen after a brutally challenging lysis of adhesions or fistula takedown, gently returning any eviscerated contents to their anatomic position in the belly. If everything has gone well, no one will ever see the surgeon's handiwork ever again. The surgeon, who deeply understands the immediacy of success or failure, strives to do something well for its own sake.

At these higher levels of practice, surgical craftsmanship also comes from developing an intuitive sense "what feels right" based on integrating all our senses—smell, sound, sight, feel, and intuition—until we act almost unconsciously. This procedural knowledge is under constant development from the earliest days of training through the last days of one's career. As we become more clinically proficient, as our breadth of exposure to all the variants of pathophysiology builds over time, our declarative "book" knowledge serves as a scaffold for procedural knowledge. In other words, as we touch and handle tissue and understand though our hands how these materials behave, we evolve beyond simply imagining Netter's illustrations superimposed on a body. In its stead, we develop a more complete and nuanced understanding of anatomy as it functions in space. As we encounter perioperative complications when the patient "did not read the textbook," our clinical decision-making tree grows more intricate branches.

Rose, Crawford, and their contemporaries argue that delineating above the neck (mind) work from below the neck (body) work is artificial and that white-collar and blue-collar labels cheapen the true value of working with one's hands. When production of cars or chairs or other handicrafts are automated, the centuries of craft honed by the "cognitively rich" interplay between hands and mind might be lost. Consequently, Rose writes, "The way work gets defined has huge material consequences—and social and civic consequences, as well." Surgeon Elliot Cutler, writing in 1929, encountered a similar idea, highlighting a period of minimal advancement in surgical sciences between the time of Galen and Ambroise Paré:

> Let them recall what happened to science for a thousand years when practice was neglected. Then will the art receive full and just credit for its share in the progress of human knowledge. [8]

The modern surgeon is both a reflection of and an exception to the white-collar/blue-collar model of work. On one hand, intellectually, a surgeon recognizes that the craft is not merely about the technical steps of an operation but requires the application of a deep understanding of anatomy, physiology, and general clinical judgment. On the other hand, the working surgeon is still beholden to base realities: our bodies are subject to physical strains, stresses, and injuries, we face labor shortages, and the quality of our work is (justly) scrutinized.

When considering a surgeon as a craftsperson honing a practical art, is it false humility to think of ourselves in part as blue-collar physicians? Historical evidence would suggest otherwise. Indeed, the origin of the word "surgeon" comes from the Greek *cheir* (hand) and *ergon* (work). In this next section, we explore the history of surgery and how our field evolved from a craft into an art.

6.1.2 Historical Perspective

The story of surgery as a craft is one of competing tensions between society, the individual craftsperson, and the field itself. In discussing this dynamic three-body relationship between creativity, craftsperson, and society, Csikszentmihalyi summarizes, "Every field is embedded in a specific social system" [6]. In other words, advancements in how we interact with the world are subject to the behaviors of dominant thought both within the field and outside of it. Think, for example, of the heliocentric model of the solar system: this model had been proposed by the ancient Greeks, fifth- and sixth-century Indian astronomers, tenth-century Islamic astronomers, and most famously by Copernicus in 1543. But until dominant societal norms changed, the theory was considered blasphemous.

Analogously, stigma toward laying one's hands on a diseased body was embedded in societal dogma throughout many major world cultures. Of course, before germ theory or antisepsis, these otherwise superstitious beliefs were lifesaving. Although the procedural skills and education levels of surgeons ebbed and flowed as knowledge was gained and lost throughout history, the common throughline of surgeon as craftsperson persisted. Indeed, the practice of surgery, which called for the handling of diseased persons with mostly bare hands, remained a job for a skilled worker from a non-elite class.

Texts as old as the code of Hammurabi contain references to laborer-physicians who would use sharp tools for wound drainage, bloodletting, circumcision, and ear lobe puncturing (including punishments for surgical complications):

> If a physician make a large incision with an operating knife and cure it, or if he open a tumor (over the eye) with an operating knife, and saves the eye, he shall receive ten shekels in money.
>
> If a physician make a large incision with the operating knife, and kill him, or open a tumor with the operating knife, and cut out the eye, his hands shall be cut off.
>
> If he had opened a tumor with the operating knife, and put out his eye, he shall pay half his value. [9]

Two millennia later, Greco-Roman surgical craftsmen would draw on prior Egyptian texts that, as the historian Ira Rutkow notes, were a "peculiar blend of superstition, ceremony, and rational thinking." This is perhaps a sentiment that even present-day surgeons will recognize.

The second-century writings of the Greek physician Galen would come to define the next 1300 years of Western medicine. Galen's instructions on surgery are pragmatic, detailing procedural steps and necessary instrumentation, and imploring the student of the healing arts to become first an expert on anatomy through observation and dissection. Compared to his treatises on physiology, which were based in experimentation, higher-level thinking, and observation, Galen treated surgery with the language of hands-on manipulation:

> All operations in surgery fall under two heads, separation and approximation. Approximation has to do with the reduction and dressing of fractures, reduction and dislocation of the joints, reductions of prolapsed intestines, uterus, or rectum, sutures of the abdomen and restoration of tissue deficiencies...Division is concerned with simple incisions, circumcisions, elevations of skin, scalping, excisions of veins, amputations, cauterization, scraping, smoothing, excisions with the saw.

Of physicians from the East, Sushruta (c.a. 800–700 BC) is thought to be the most learned practitioner of surgery. Unlike his Western contemporaries, he regarded surgery as the "highest in value," with the "superior advantage of producing instantaneous effects by means of surgical instruments and appliances." His comments echo the same exaltations of flow states and immediacy discussed earlier. In his collected writings, the *Samhita Sushruta* describes stunningly modern ideas, including using fruits, vegetables, and animal specimens for simulation and practice for incisions, excisions, drainage, cautery, enemas, and ligaturing. Remarkably, Sushruta also describes techniques for antisepsis as well as complex operations including laparotomy, intestinal repair, lithotomy, herniorrhaphy, amputation, cesarean section, cataract treatment, and rhinoplasty. He implores his students, "Only the union of medicine and surgery constitutes the complete doctor."

Returning to West over a millennium later, the age of the barber-surgeon may be regarded as a dark and curious period in the history of surgery. However, barber-surgeons served as stewards of early surgical technique, passing down the craft from father to son. They continued to perform herniorrhaphy, bladder stone extraction, and treatment of cataracts, refining their craft over the course of generations. They did the job of medical doctors at lower cost, and Rutkow notes that "surgeons tended to be comparable in social status to the artisans, the middle and lower classes, and the small-scale merchants, who made up a much greater portion of the populace than the wealthy patients of the Paris physicians." Subdivisions in medical versus surgical practice would continue to become even more confusing in twelfth through fifteenth century Europe. In France, three separate groups existed: barber-surgeons, an "academic enclave" of surgeons, and itinerant surgeons or "cutters." Practice encroachment was a constant source of tension, culminating with both guilds of barber-surgeons and academic surgeons lobbying university medical faculty for partnership. In the thirteenth century, the French surgeon Lanfranc expresses his frustration with these separations, writing:

> Why is there such a great difference between surgeons and physicians? The philosophers have placed the craft in the hands of laymen, for many disdain to work with their hands; and many think it is impossible for one person to know both medicine and surgery. But know this well, that no man can be a good physician who knows no surgery; and conversely, no one can be a good surgeon without knowledge of medicine.

Perhaps the most notable craftsman in the barber-surgeon's guild was Ambroise Paré. From humble beginnings as the son of a cabinetmaker, he reached the height of academic success, and his surgical textbooks, written in vernacular French instead of Latin, were taught in medical schools within his lifetime. Paré played a pivotal role in turning contemporary practitioners away from the philosophies of ancient surgeons. Instead, he wrote volumes of methodical observations drawn from during countless hours of training and practice. As an army surgeon, Paré learned and wrote about ligation rather than cautery for hemorrhage control during amputation. Although orchiectomy during herniorrhaphy was common and accepted during that time, Paré found that it was unnecessary and argued against the practice. He devised surgical instruments and hernia truss belts. He even contributed significantly to advances in dental care.

It would take another 100 years for European surgeons to be elevated from the ranks of "technicians or craftsmen" to a social status comparable to that of physicians. In a retrospective view, one might observe that key surgeons pushed for two simultaneous movements: the first was a movement toward scientific observation and knowledge of anatomy and away from superstition and ancient theorems; the second was a movement away from itinerant practitioners without accountability and toward governing licensing bodies. The elevation of the field back into the ranks of medicine was perhaps less deliberate and more attributable to society's inability to deny the importance of the craft of surgery in treating illness. An upward shift in social status impacted the structure of surgical education, with techniques for operations, research, and anatomy being taught in schools as opposed to merely by apprenticeship [10, 11].

A particular feature of early American exceptionalism is that physicians in post-colonial America were wholly different from those in Europe, with no defined separation between physicians and surgeons. This persisted until the nearly turn of the twentieth century: all American physicians were general practitioners who could perform surgery with little to no additional required training. This changed with the founding of the American Surgical Association in 1880 under the leadership of Dr. Samuel Gross, famously depicted in a painting by Thomas Eakins (a favorite of textbook publishers). Around this time, William Halsted would impose his pyramidal surgical training program at Johns Hopkins, the rigor of which would inform general surgical training programs through to current paradigms. In the early twentieth century, the growing demand for well-trained surgeons was evident. The pyramidal model, based on an arguably archaic apprenticeship model, produced very few master surgeons and far more incompletely trained surgeons, echoing a time in Europe when itinerant surgeons could fill gaps in care with variable success (or failure). Thus, in 1939, Dr. Edward Churchill instated the "rectangular" five-plus-two residency model that has persisted through the current era [11].

Even as the art and science of surgery has continued to evolve, the hands of the modern surgeon seem to remember the spirit of innovation and manual competence of the barber-surgeons of history. For instance, the first laparoscopic cholecystectomy was performed in 1987 when a surgeon, Dr. Philippe Mouret, was asked if he could remove the gallbladder at the time of pelvic adhesiolysis. The patient had been suffering from symptomatic cholelithiasis. At first, Mouret refused, as laparoscopy was only typically used for gynecologic cases. But by the end of the index operation, he simply turned his instruments cephalad and excised the gallbladder without much difficulty or fanfare. As a craftsman, the surgeon demonstrated obvious technical expertise and comfort with his instruments, a clear understanding of anatomy, intuition about the feasibility of the procedure, scientific curiosity, and empathy toward a suffering patient [12].

What comes next for surgeon craftsperson? We seem to be constantly approaching an inflection point of technological progress that threatens to subsume the human element of any craft. Will artificial intelligence imitate our abilities well enough to make the human surgeon obsolete? We should be cautious of any technology that asks us to divest in the tradition of craftsmanship for the benefit of efficiency—as error is reduced, so is nuance and connection. In the next section, we explore the human touch that gives our craft its artistic nature.

6.2 Surgery as Art

> Tell us please, what treatment in an emergency is administered by ear?
>
> I met his gaze and I did not blink. "Words of comfort," I said to my father. (Abraham Verghese, MD, *Cutting for Stone* [13])

In the previous section, we posed that surgery has intrinsic artistic value as a craft. But the art of surgery obviously extends beyond the tip of a scalpel or the red line of the operating room. What does it take to develop deep and trusting relationships with our patients? How do we lead teams in and out of the operating room? Can we develop our own personal approach to patient care while abiding by the rules of physiology and the economic realities of modern medicine? The nontechnical "soft" skills such as empathy, integrity, communication styles, intraoperative problem-solving, and appropriate patient selection, all are critical.

This argument might seem to negate the importance of surgery as a "craft." Instead, however, we propose that if the nucleus of the "Art of Surgery" is dedication to craft, the surrounding electrons are the soft skills in their various valence orbitals, inexorably related to each other as a single element. Put another way, the musician who practices their instrument for 10,000 hours may still perform the same piece differently at Carnegie Hall or in a subway station—dedication to their craft occurs in the practice room, but the application of the art is learned through engagement with their audiences and environments.

Similarly, the nontechnical skills that fill out the art of surgery are built around variety and unpredictability: a unique patient encounter that stays with us for a lifetime, the words of wisdom from a colleague that come to us at exactly the right time, and the ways we interact with the ever-changing teams we work with.

In this section, we rely on a teleological approach to exploring this complex concept, approaching the art of surgery by examining its result, rather than by the means. As noted earlier, this relates to what Polyani refers to as "tacit knowledge," in which the only evidence of that a skill exists is the result this skill produces. He writes, "Rules of art can be useful, but they do not determine the practice of an art; they are maxims which can serve as a guide to the art only if they can be integrated into the practical knowledge of the art. They cannot replace this knowledge" [14].

Similarly, the outcome of what we do as surgeons is simply inherent to every decision we make. In this framework, the art of surgery might be understood as the many behaviors that inform the way we ease a patient's suffering—that there is no one way to define it, but that we know what it is when we see it.

In his 1951 book, *The Philosophy of Surgery,* vascular surgeon Rene Leriche wrote:

> The art of operating is possible in part by habit, skills add a bit of excellence on top and everyone can achieve this art within a very short time. However, performing surgery in the right place and at the right time, knowing when it is necessary or if it can be avoided, the conditions that effect success or failure, the changes of plan in surgery based on these conditions, the outcome to be expected and the means to obtaining these results as much as possible: These are the difficult aspects of the art of surgery and the elements that constitute its science. [15, 16]

The evolution of patient autonomy provides us with excellent illustration of surgery as an artform in progress. Take, for example, the cases of two very different patients. The first might be a woman with a complex recurrent incisional hernia related to a prior lower midline cesarean section. The problem may not be life-threatening, and the patient may simply be looking for a technical fix so she can move on with her life. But before even meeting the patient, the surgeon knows simply from the diagnosis that a redo incisional hernia operation will be technically challenging, will require careful application of years of training, and will be physically grueling. An array of postoperative complications to be avoided instantaneously pops into the surgeon's mind. The gap between the patient and surgeon's understanding of the problem seems as vast as a desert expanse, with the eventual goal of the operating room appearing to be a far-off oasis somewhere in between. Therefore, to find a way to the operating room in the first place, the surgeon might first query the patient's perspectives: when did she first notice the hernia? What impact has this condition had on her ability to work or care for her family? What would be an acceptable quality of life? What is her understanding of the ways in which her life may or may not change after surgery? Who will help her in the days after the operation? What is her current state of health? What can she do to prepare herself so that she can have the best outcome after surgery?

Of course, not every case requires quite this level of deep understanding of the patient. But to some degree, in even the most minor procedure, the boldness required to take a scalpel to fellow human requires us to somehow package our technical competence into a projection of a practitioner worthy of trust. In his 2001 presidential address to the New England Surgical Society, Dr. H. David Crombie said:

> Incising into the body of another human being carries with it a sense of responsibility and awe that does not grow larger or smaller with the extent of the procedure. It exists in each case to its fullest. When do we perceive it? When do we acquire this sense of awe that prompts our asking for consent and expressing sorrow for loss?

Dr. Crombie goes on to describe an experience he had with one of his own patients, the second of the patients in our example. The patient was a 75-year-old woman with metastatic ovarian cancer causing recurrent small bowel obstructions who had been referred to him for a gastrostomy so that she could be freed of her nasogastric tube. "The procedure was helpful," he states. "With the tube-to-gravity drainage, she was able to enjoy the tastes and flavors of small feedings of liquids, custards, and ice cream... One morning on my rounds after she related her pleasure at a few tasty swallows, I noticed a large, hardbound book as big as an encyclopedia on her bedside table. The title: The Collected Works of Emily Dickinson." Dr. Crombie finds out that in her weakened state, his patient cannot read the hardcover book in bed because it is too heavy, so he brings her a paperback anthology. The next day, she requests him to read aloud the poems she wanted him to see, including the pithy entry, "Surgeons must be very careful When they take the knife! Underneath their fine incisions Stirs the culprit—Life!" Reflecting on this experience years later, Dr. Crombie relates:

> There I was, early in my surgical career, groomed for competitiveness in college, medical school, and residency, trained to be a decisive surgeon, and I was being called on to ease the pain of dying by reading poetry to a 75-year-old woman. [17]

Dr. Crombie's experience feels familiar—how do we reconcile appreciation for the handicraft of the work with the art of shouldering the responsibility for a fragile human life? Dr. Lisa Rosenbaum captures this tension inherent to surgical practice in her essay entitled "Beyond Moral Injury—Can We Reclaim Agency, Belief, and Joy in Medicine?" She recounts a story she found on social media during the COVID-19 pandemic, in which a chief resident describes a busy morning seeing several new patients. One patient cannot give the resident an accurate history because she is too upset about having forgotten her favorite candy at home. Late in the day, just before sign-out time, the resident returns to the patient's room with a box of that candy. Dr. Rosenbaum writes, "Although the Milk Duds kept [the resident] at the hospital far longer than intended (her patient suddenly opened up), for the first time that day she felt her work had meaning. So she wondered: What if improving our own well-being sometimes means spending more time at work rather than less?" [18].

In Rosenbaum's telling, the resident has just uncovered that perfect equilibrium point between technical skill acquisition and the skills of a nurturing, caring physician that can only be learned at the patient's bedside—she has found flow outside of the operating room. Reaching a state of flow in a nontechnical setting is therefore possible, especially for surgeons. Csikszentmihalyi writes, "The best moments in our lives are not the passive, receptive, relaxing times…The best moments usually occur if a person's body or mind is stretched to its limits in a voluntary effort to accomplish something difficult and worthwhile." Striking this balance is challenging: we know that technical skills seem to diminish after a certain point beyond which fatigue and stress take over, but soft skills may increase with more dedicated time at the bedside. We can learn so much through the moments spent simply listening to a patient tell their story, uninterrupted, but we risk violating or duty-hour restrictions or delaying already packed clinic days.

In search of flow, we are often stretched to our limits of fatigue, with sleep and other bodily functions easily ignored. Extraneous noise from the outside world and internal chatter falls away. When this happens, surgeons may find themselves in a liminal space, where there is no separation between self and the task at hand, and all decisions are made in the interest of caring for the whole patient at the deepest physical level—the depths of flesh, as well as a deep spiritual level—the depths of trust. Ultimately, tackling the difficult task becomes second nature. Even when complications arise, the surgeon draws on the strength of the relationship with the patient and their family to proceed forward.

6.2.1 Innovation

A primary definition of "art" is that it is inherently creative. We have now explored surgery as craft, surgery as history, and surgery for its intangible soft skills. But what of surgery as a creative art form? Surely, very few patients would come to see us asking us to invent an operation to cure what ails them. But innovation and continuous improvement are essential to our field—recall the daring innovations of Paré or Alexis Carrel or, more recently, surgeons who continue to push the boundaries of our craft through fewer and smaller incisions.

How do surgeons innovate and create while respecting the boundaries of our ethical obligations to the patient? How do we abandon old dogmas in search of new frontiers? Once again, Csikszentmihalyi suggests an answer: we are problem finders. Surgeons innovate through necessity, understanding the gap between what can be done and what needs to be done. The greatest creative minds among us are often the ones who simply work the most and have been exposed to every challenge (including failure); they have been exposed to unusual stimuli outside of our field; they listen to silence and observe the negative space to understand what is missing; they see potential. As we have already seen, the innovation does not always necessarily need to be accompanied by any fanfare: the surgeon may simply turn the laparoscope from pelvis to right upper quadrant and change the fundamental direction of surgical progress forever.

When surgeons stay curious and find problems, we find ourselves collaborating with engineers (robotics, endovascular) and bench scientists (xenotransplant), with astronauts (aerospace surgery) and glassblowers (fiberoptic endoscopy). We employ our soft skills in team leadership and communication to arrive at these new heights together. We use our aesthetic judgment to understand when a new creation "looks right."

Surgeons who actively search for these negative spaces play in the arena of visual artists, musicians, dancers, and writers—creatives who see potential in blank pages and empty space. Musicians from Mozart to Miles Davis are quoted as defining their music by the spaces *between* the notes. In this sense, every patient interaction, every operation, and every mundane postoperative order is an opportunity to find potential for creative expression—a well-honed prehabilitation plan, a smooth and efficient case, a moment at the bedside that reveals something personal about your patient you didn't know before [19–21].

6.3 Conclusion

Perhaps all attempts to precisely describe the Art of Surgery are like trying to gaze at a very faint star in the night sky, which is only observable when your eyes are slightly averted. E.B. White once wrote, "Humor can be dissected, as a frog can, but the thing dies in the process and the innards are discouraging to any but the purely scientific mind." Earlier we described the art of surgery as an impressionist painting, but perhaps the more we explore this concept, the more we risk "dissecting the frog."

No matter how we cut it, we have all felt the deep fulfillment of life when we practice the Art of Surgery. But to preserve this fulfillment for generations of future physicians, we need to ensure that the intrinsically enjoyable aspects of our profession are accentuated and not suppressed. As the future of medicine continues to develop, deep introspection can help us identify the core values we rely on in practice, whether that is the quality of time spent with patients, the relationships we develop with our mentors, the ability to become an expert in an operation, or, conversely, the freedom to broaden our scope and innovate. We can continue to explore the Art of Surgery even when the economic pressures of healthcare continue to bear down, and while our dedication to these core values may well strain the vice, this pushback might be necessary.

In the middle of the last century, Leriche presciently wrote:

> Maybe one day in the future such a time will come that the surgeon will perform surgery on a patient who he did not examine personally, the art will fall into a simple performance situation, so technique, inevitably, will become superior to therapeutics. [14]

One can almost detect Leriche's sadness at the thought of a surgeon as a pure technician. Indeed, he later stated, "The danger of forgetting the human, who are in the target beyond their humor, consisting of flesh and sense... Each surgeon should be a equipped with the deepest respect for the human being." [14].

As technology continues to evolve, we continue to worry about the encroachment of artificial intelligence or other automated systems into our lives, removing the autonomy of our art. The threat is certainly real. However, we pose that by appreciating the finer points of the art of our field, we can have agency over how we invite and use technology to enhance our practice. For instance, a surgical robot can enhance precision; image-guidance reduces the cognitive burden of uncertainty; large language model-based artificial intelligence can summarize stacks of patient records, allowing us to spend more time in face-to-face patient care.

Whatever the future brings, it is clear that surgery is and should remain inherently artistic. At its core, it is work of manual dexterity and craft, of skill and grace, of practice and performance, of aesthetics and precision. It is enveloped in dedication, compassion, curiosity, and intellectual flexibility. It reflects strength and fragility, persistence in the face of all breaking points, resilience through failure. The art of surgery is the qualia of what we feel it to be when we practice it day in and day out.

References

1. Rose M. The mind at work: valuing the intelligence of the American worker. New York: Penguin Books; 2005.
2. Dennett DC. Quining qualia. In: Marcel A, Bisiach E, editors. Consciousness in modern science. Oxford: Oxford University Press; 1988. Reprinted in: Lycan W, editor. Mind and

cognition: a reader. Cambridge: MIT Press; 1990. Also in: Goldman A, editor. Readings in philosophy and cognitive science. Cambridge: MIT Press; 1993.
3. Qualia (Stanford Encyclopedia of Philosophy). [Internet]. 2021 Aug 12. Available from: https://plato.stanford.edu/Entries/qualia/#Uses. Accessed 26 May 2024.
4. Bass BL. Our lives as surgeons: finding a sense of place and purpose. J Am Coll Surg. 2015;220(5):790–6. https://doi.org/10.1016/j.jamcollsurg.2015.01.003.
5. Crawford MB. Shop class as soulcraft. The New Atlantis. 2006;13:7–24.
6. Csikszentmihalyi M. The systems model of creativity: the collected works of Mihaly Csikszentmihalyi. 1st ed. Dordrecht: Springer; 2014.
7. Csikszentmihalyi M. Flow: the psychology of optimal experience. 1st Harper Perennial Modern Classics ed. New York: Harper Perennial; 2008.
8. Cutler EC. The art of surgery. Arch Surg. 1929;18(4):1190–9. https://doi.org/10.1001/archsurg.1929.01140130280013.
9. Halwani T, Takrouri M. Medical laws and ethics of Babylon as read in Hammurabi's code (History). Int J Law Healthc Ethics. 2006;4(2). https://www.academia.dk/MedHist/Biblioteket/Print/hamurabi-medical-laws-and-ethics-of-babylon.html
10. Rutkow I. Surgery: an illustrated history. St. Louis: Mosby-Year Book Inc.; 1993.
11. Camison L, Brooker JE, Naran S, Potts JR III, Losee JE. The history of surgical education in the United States: past, present, and future. Ann Surg Open. 2022;3(1) https://doi.org/10.1097/AS9.0000000000000148.
12. Bismuth H. Discovery and innovation in surgery: chance and necessity. Ann Surg. 2021;274(5):688–9.
13. Verghese A. Cutting for stone: a novel. New York: Alfred A. Knopf; 2009.
14. Polanyi M. Personal knowledge: towards a post-critical philosophy. London: Routledge; 2002 [1958].
15. Leriche R. La Philosophie de la Chirurgie. Paris: Flammarion; 1951.
16. Akça T, Aydın S. René Leriche and "philosophy of surgery" in the light of contemporary medical ethics. Ulus Cerrahi Derg. 2013;29(3):131–8. https://doi.org/10.5152/UCD.2013.2248. PMID: 25931863; PMCID: PMC4379813.
17. Crombie HD. The surgeon's art. Arch Surg. 2002;137(4):390–6. https://doi.org/10.1001/archsurg.137.4.390.
18. Rosenbaum L. Beyond moral injury: can we reclaim agency, belief, and joy in medicine? N Engl J Med. 2024;390:951.
19. The Decision Lab. Adaptive control of thought. [Internet]. 2021. Available from: https://thedecisionlab.com/reference-guide/neuroscience/adaptive-control-of-thought. Accessed 1 Apr 2024.
20. Bolwerk A, Mack-Andrick J, Lang FR, Dörfler A, Maihöfner C. How art changes your brain: differential effects of visual art production and cognitive art evaluation on functional brain connectivity. PLoS One 2014;9(7). https://doi.org/10.1371/journal.pone.0101035. PMID: 24983951; PMCID: PMC4077746.
21. Austin L. Perspective: problem finding and the multidisciplinary mind. Science. 2009 February 20; Available from: https://www.science.org/content/article/perspective-problem-finding-and-multidisciplinary-mind

Chapter 7
Applied Ethics in Surgery: What Do We Invite Patients to Trust?

Marguerite W. Spruce, Vishal G. Shelat, Kyler Squirrell, Douglas Brown, and Piroska Kopar

7.1 Introduction

To trust is to be sufficiently confident in the integrity (e.g., truth, ability, reliability) of a subject/object to participate in an action that includes personal risk. It is a pivotal aspect of all facets of life, and healthcare demands exceptional trust because of its critical consequences. Furthermore, surgery requires a special level of trust because of its invasive nature and its practice under anesthesia when patients are perhaps most vulnerable. From where does this trust originate? And what are its limits?

To answer these questions, one must closely examine the relationship(s) in which the trust exists. While not a complete list, three prominent relationships are key to understanding trust—i.e., (1) the physician/surgeon and the patient, (2) the physician/surgeon and other medical providers/institutions, and (3) the physician/surgeon and society. The phrase "social contract" is often used to describe a mutual agreement between the medical profession and society, but the phrase has been hotly debated in recent years amidst the rapidly changing medical field and the world at large.

In this chapter, we examine the most pressing ethical concerns of surgical practice today, which include but are certainly not limited to (1) the loss of trust in science and the medical community, (2) enduring disparities in healthcare, (3) increased specialization with care fragmentation, (4) the rise of shift work that has altered the patient-physician relationship, (5) the push for a more consumer-merchant approach to surgery, and (6) political interference/loss of self-regulation. We utilize case scenarios to analyze the implications of these trends and evaluate them through a humanistic lens. This lens allows us to focus our "responsibility to lead ethical lives

M. W. Spruce · V. G. Shelat · K. Squirrell · D. Brown · P. Kopar (✉)
Center for Humanism and Ethics in Surgical Specialties, Washington University, St. Louis, MO, USA
e-mail: pkopar@wustl.edu

F. Jotterand, C. Bosco (eds.), *Fostering Humanism in Surgery*, New Paradigms in Healthcare, https://doi.org/10.1007/978-3-031-82771-6_7

of personal fulfillment that aspire to the greater good" [1] which centers on the reasoning as well as the dignity, personal experience, and potential of the individual [1]. We then associate these current conflicts with the historical social contract as a way to evaluate its place in this rapidly changing world. We first look more closely into the history of the social contract and medicine as a profession.

7.2 The Social Contract

Medical care has evolved over time, yet healers have held an important place in societies for as long as records are available. In the past, healers were independent, diverse, unregulated, and often intertwined with sorcery. Today medicine is considered to be a profession (i.e., "a paid occupation, especially one that involves prolonged training and a formal qualification" [2]). Most credit Hippocrates, a Greek physician and philosopher, with the origin of medicine viewed as a profession, pointing to the famous Hippocratic Oath [3]. This tradition established standards of conduct for physicians based on empirical observation [3, 4]. However, these standards were not universally accepted or practiced, and the standardization of medical education did not begin until the Middle Ages.

During plague outbreaks, doctors were urged to remain with and care for infected individuals as opposed to the accepted practice of leaving with the goal of self-preservation [4]. Using the phrase "medical ethics" to describe what physicians ought to do did not emerge until the early nineteenth century in English physician Thomas Percival's 1803 book *Medical Ethics* [4, 5]. However, such attempts to define social obligations for physicians were not yet widely adopted. Instead, it was assumed that a written code was unnecessary for a gentleman whose good character was sufficient. Just over 40 years later, the American Medical Association (AMA) published the 1847 *Code of Medical Ethics*, the first national code of ethics. This code was born out of necessity in the United States, as there were no uniform standards for the education or practice of medicine, and trust in the English tradition of "gentlemanliness" without a written contract was low after the Revolutionary War [4].

The AMA's *Code of Medical Ethics* and the establishment of licensing laws [4, 6] created medicine's social contract or the medical community's unwritten contract with the society it served. The foundation of this contract was professionalism [6], which required a set of standard ethics, morals, and behavior. The basis of the contract was trust. The contract covered three separate but overlapping relationships: physicians and patients, physicians and other physicians, and physicians and their communities [4].

In this code, physicians' behavior was to be based on a deontological understanding of right and wrong. In every action, they were expected to act in the best interest of their patients, the medical community, and society. Physicians were expected to be "ever ready," [7] both physically and mentally, to care for their patients. They were expected to be polite, virtuous, and sincere with a focus on patient confidentiality. They were expected to sacrifice their own comfort, ease, and health for the welfare of their patients [7]. In return, patients were expected to be honest and concise, obey doctors' orders, and show appreciation.

The AMA code obligated physicians to "maintain the highest purity of character and standards of moral excellence" [7]. They were to cover for one another, maintain respect in consultations, and avoid self-promotion [7]. Additionally, physicians were called to serve the community in addition to individual patients. They were to be "ever ready to give counsel to the public" [7] and to face danger "for the alleviation of the suffering, even at the jeopardy of their own lives" [7]. They were responsible for protecting the integrity of their profession by exposing "quacks." In return, the public was to maintain the utmost respect for physicians and properly discern "true science" [7]. There were additional implicit societal expectations regarding physicians—e.g., autonomy, trust, monopoly, status and rewards, and self-regulation [8].

One can see that some of these expectations remain prominent today whereas others are not. The first revision of the AMA code in 1903 eliminated the written obligations of patients and society and focused solely on the expectations of physicians [9]. The most recent update—introduced in 2016—reiterates many of the common themes of compassion, respect, professionalism, and competence as well as reporting colleagues who are not upholding these standards. This revision includes the expectations of continuing medical education and advancement as well as supporting "access to medical care for all people" [10]. Physicians do have the right, though, to choose their patients outside of emergency situations.

The AMA code has never been a steadfast and unchanging document but rather a fluid document that has been revised at least seven times since its original publication [9]. The need for edits has arisen for many reasons, the foremost being rapid medical advancements which have given rise to today's most pressing ethical concerns in surgery.

7.3 Today's Pressing Ethical Concerns

The Information Age has led to the transformation of the field of medicine in numerous ways. First, the widespread dissemination of information and misinformation, along with many other factors, has led to an erosion of trust in the medical community [11]. Rapid advancements have led to increased specialization, shift work, and a demand for a consumer-merchant relationship. These changes—which have highlighted and perhaps exacerbated severe disparities—have occurred with a lack of medical involvement in policy-making. The social contract has been strained as a result, with some arguing that it has fractured [3, 4, 8, 10]. The following case example illustrates the complex interplay of multiple dimensions of holistic, person-centered healthcare delivery with emphasis on ethical issues.

Case 1

Patient A, a 48- year-old patient with a history of sickle cell anemia, is admitted to the intensive care unit (ICU) after a motor vehicle collision with numerous injuries, including right-sided rib fractures with air and blood in the chest cavity, significant liver laceration, and right lower extremity fractures. Following the operative repair of his right leg fractures, he develops low blood pressure from surgical blood loss requiring blood transfusion. He then develops sickle cell crisis with hyper-hemolysis (red blood cell death), which is further complicated by multiorgan failure. After being sedated and placed on a ventilator, his sister becomes his surrogate medical decision-maker. Despite aggressive medical care, his condition continues to decline.

The ICU provider meets with his sister and other family members to discuss Patient A's worsening clinical status. The family explains that they are from Rwanda and have a strong Christian faith whereby they believe that God will heal him and that choosing any avenue short of maximal medical therapy will equate to a lack of faith. They express frustration with the patient's worsening clinical status and think it is the result of negligence. They also believe that he is receiving substandard care because of his race, including feeling pushed to "pull the plug." The ICU provider attempts to dissuade these beliefs, but these concerns remain. Regarding the new onset of acute liver failure, the hepatology team explains that liver transplant will not be offered because of his sickle cell disease, as the risk of transplanted liver failure would be too high. This decision exacerbates the family's belief that Patient A's race is impacting the medical team's decisions. Despite ongoing aggressive care, he continues to decompensate. Blood transfusion is reserved for life-threatening shock, as it could accelerate hyper-hemolysis. This development begins to occur at increasing frequency, with ongoing multisystem organ failure.

Pain medications and sedatives are held to monitor for improvement in mental status, as requested by the family, but the team becomes concerned about their patient's discomfort and futility, particularly with ongoing usage of blood products. The care team reports being called "racist" by the family and having their conversations recorded. The family continues to desire full measures, including cardiopulmonary resuscitation (CPR) in the event of a cardiac arrest.

Case 1 Preliminary Ethical Assessment

Patient A has multiorgan failure with minimal medical options beyond the intensive care he is currently receiving. Numerous physicians have determined that further care, including blood transfusion and CPR, is non-beneficial. His healthcare team has also expressed concern for inadequate treatment of his pain, which was directly requested to be withheld by his family. His sister is his surrogate decision-maker but may no longer be acting in his best interest, raising concerns about her suitability as such.

7.3.1 Erosion of Trust

The foundation of the social contract is professionalism, and the foundation of professionalism is trust [12]. In Patient A's case, we see a fractured trust. Trust in the American medical system has been on the decline since the 1970s [11]. Interestingly, trust is highest for individual practitioners, lower for hospital systems, and lowest for health insurance and pharmaceutical companies [11]. This decline in trust has mirrored the decline in trust in the government as a whole, and the causes are multifactorial [11].

First, medical information is no longer a commodity held by select individuals but rather is widely and freely accessible online. Expanding access to medical information has resulted in a reconfiguration of patients' need for physicians and a growing tendency for patients to challenge their physicians on specific subjects discovered through independent (re)search. It has also led to the dissemination of both misinformation and disinformation, which most patients have trouble discerning. The public health consequences are significant (e.g., lower vaccination rates) [13].

Second, numerous high-profile examples of poor ethical practices by physicians and the larger medical system have contributed to an erosion of trust. Well-known incidents include the Tuskegee experiments and Nuremberg trials [5] as well as the practice of racially segregated medical care in the United States [14]. There continues to be a larger deficit in trust in the medical system within communities of color, the origin of which is not solely the result of atrocities of the past. Ongoing, everyday racism—whether personal or structural, subtle or overt, intentional or not—further erodes trust [15].

Patient A's case illustrates how our familiar approach to ethical dilemmas can be inadequate if we fail to acknowledge and address cultural differences. The task of rebuilding trust is comprehensive and beyond the scope of this chapter, but we propose that the rebuilding can start with individual patient encounters. Doctors who show genuine care and concern, avoid medical jargon, provide adequate time, and create an atmosphere for patients and families to share their concerns can help regain their patients' trust. In addition, research has shown that trust increases when patients have providers who look like them [14]. When this visual familiarity is not possible, perhaps involving other caregivers with similar appearance and/or cultural background can be impactful in establishing trust. Providers must be cognizant of their biases, acknowledge their limitations especially when caring for patients with different backgrounds from their own, and ask for help. However, it is essential to recognize that trust alone cannot resolve the deeper issues at play; the systemic disparities in health outcomes must also be addressed to ensure equity in patient care.

7.3.2 Healthcare Disparities

Health disparities are differences in the "attainment of full health potential" among specific groups of people [16] that result from unjust and often deep-rooted systemic inequalities. These health inequities exist along the entire spectrum of life, from gestational age to chronic medical illnesses, homicide-related death, and life expectancy [16]. In the United States, disparities exist based on race and ethnicity, geographic location, age, gender, socioeconomic status, sexual orientation, and many more demographic variables [16].

Most physicians in the United States have formally pledged to treat their patients with justice, regardless of background. Yet, competing or conflicting priorities within the modern healthcare system make doing so difficult, if not impossible. Additional parties have been added to the social contract—e.g., large hospital systems, insurance companies, pharmaceutical companies, and medical device companies. While pharmaceutical and medical device companies have introduced dramatic advances in what we can offer patients, these advances also have come at a premium that not everyone can afford. This sobering reality has, in part, given rise to the massive differences in what providers can provide. Physicians may tailor their prescribing practices to what (if any) insurance coverage someone has. They may offer a lower quality implant or orthotic because the patient cannot afford it and/or the physical therapy it would require. They see patients present at later stages of disease or with preventable complications due to disparate geographic location or socioeconomic status. They watch young people die of gun violence. Such repeated experiences lead to moral injury, which "describes the challenge of simultaneously knowing what care patients need but being unable to provide it due to constraints that are beyond our control" [17]. This moral injury leads eventually to moral crisis among healthcare providers, the endpoint of which is burnout.

Within the medical system, physicians must take some responsibility for the erosion of trust. Physicians are guilty of holding and even acting with prejudice. There are numerous historical cases of explicit bias, including but certainly not limited to the atrocities committed by Nazi physicians or a history of racial segregation in the United States with enduring patterns [18, 19]. Evidence has proven that implicit bias affects how well-intentioned physicians practice medicine, thereby unwittingly exacerbating healthcare disparities [20].

Healthcare disparities not only injure our patients but also our own morality. Combating healthcare disparities may seem a daunting task, but the first step is to acknowledge our own biases [20]. We must practice individualized and trauma-informed care (TIC) [21]. TIC is a treatment framework for understanding the complex interactions and consequences of trauma to both the body and the mind. TIC emphasizes treatment that protects patients and providers from additional harm [22]. We must also work with our administrators and legislators. Healthcare providers must have a seat at the table in deciding the structure of the healthcare system to ensure that it is equitable.

Case 1 Ethical Assessment Through a Humanistic Lens

Patient A is a Black patient with a disease that largely affects people who look like him and who have been marginalized in this country, including by the medical community, for hundreds of years. Not offering transplantation because of sickle cell disease may be interpreted as direct discrimination. Determining that further blood transfusion is futile and should be withheld in part because it is a limited resource could be interpreted as placing other patients before him. He is also originally from another country with different cultural norms and religious beliefs than most of his healthcare providers. These providers could be underestimating the family's religious faith, which may be of paramount importance, including over personal comfort.

Healthcare disparities and mistrust go hand in hand. Evidence has shown that patients desire doctors who "look like them, talk like them, or share their life experiences" [15]. While we cannot look like all of our patients, we can respond to our patients and their families with empathy instead of judgment. We can also enlist colleagues or other staff members who might share certain characteristics in order to bridge the gap and reestablish trust. While the first case illustrates the issues relating to the patient and physician, next we discuss the issues relevant to the physician and peers within the healthcare system.

Case 2

Patient B, a 72-year-old patient with a history of diabetes, heart disease, and colorectal cancer with prior surgery, radiation, and chemotherapy, presents to a small community hospital at 4 a.m. on a Thursday morning with signs and symptoms of a small bowel obstruction. He undergoes an abdominal CT scan that shows an obstruction with concern for lack of blood flow to the intestine, necessitating urgent operation. The patient is known to the colorectal surgical service at the university hospital 3 hours away and has followed with their clinic ever since his diagnosis. The on-call general surgeon at the community hospital requests transfer because he is uncomfortable operating on someone with a complicated abdominal surgical history with prior cancer. Patient B continues to get sicker and arrives at the university hospital at 5 p.m., at which time the colorectal surgeons are still in the operating room with elective cases and with more operative cases on their schedules the next day. Given these conflicts and the urgency of the operation, the admitting team turns to the acute care surgery team for help. After reviewing risks and benefits of the operation, the acute care surgery team takes the patient to the operating room and finds dead intestine that is resected. His hospital course is complicated by kidney failure requiring dialysis. After 3 weeks of several other complications, his care is changed to comfort measures, and he passes away. The chief of the acute care surgery section wants to know why the colorectal service did not operate on the patient.

Case 2 Preliminary Ethical Assessment

Patient B has advanced colorectal cancer with previous treatment including surgery. His current presentation is a known complication of his disease and treatment, and the appropriate operation was offered to him after reviewing risks and benefits with him and his family in line with the principles of informed consent. However, it is possible that his complicated course and death were partially caused by a delay in care.

7.3.3 Increased Medical Specialization and Shift Work

Medicine in 1847, when the AMA *Code of Medical Ethics* was published, relied on a single family physician who managed all aspects of a patient's care, consulting others as needed. Medical knowledge has increased exponentially since that time, becoming far too great for any one practitioner to obtain and maintain. As a result, the medical community is now highly specialized, with numerous consultants involved in managing complex or critically ill patients. While this sub-specialization has advanced medical knowledge and improved outcomes for certain conditions, it has also introduced various problems.

First, care is often fragmented with poor communication among providers, leaving patients feeling lost in the shuffle. This breakdown occurs within a single hospital due to care provided by numerous teams, sometimes with conflicting recommendations. The *1847 AMA Code* laid out specific guidance for consultations, including direct communication between the primary physician and consultant prior to providing final recommendations to the patient, equal share of credit or blame for the outcome, and maintenance of mutual respect [7]. This arrangement is rarely executed, to the detriment of all stakeholders—i.e., the patient, the physicians, and the healthcare system. Trust is eroded due to actual or perceived poor communication and disrespect.

Sub-specialization and the resulting intra-institutional politics have also led to competition and conflict between specialties, as opposed to collaboration, and have contributed to the ethical complexity. For example, surgical tradition would have required Patient B's colorectal surgeon to operate on him, even if it were during late hours and even if the surgeon had to change her schedule for the following day. Assuming that she would have handled the findings and the operation in a similar way to the acute care surgery team, the outcome for the patient would have been the same for the patient. So does it matter? While the outcome may be the same for the patient, it would not be the same for several other affected parties. First, the family of Patient B may potentially trust the institution more by having continuity in Patient B's care. Second, the patient who was scheduled to have an operation with the colorectal surgeon the following day may either have the surgery rescheduled or performed by a sleep-deprived surgeon with possible effects on the outcome. Third, the colorectal surgeon may have increased her own mortality rates—a figure that is reported publicly with increasing frequency—a consequence that could impact her standing amongst peers as well as potentially lead to loss of repute with its repercussions. Fourth, the hospital would almost certainly have lost money by providing prolonged ICU care to Patient B, and this loss would have counted against the section of colorectal surgery rather than the section of acute care surgery. In a department of surgery in which limited resources are divided among sections according to the generation of revenue, this implication has consequences for respective patient populations and health equity.

While shift work has many advantages to both patients and providers, it has also contributed to the degradation of the physician-patient relationship and potentially even the professional status of the surgeon. Operations not completed during routine business hours are often passed to the on-call surgeon, whether within the surgeon's own team or from another service, as we saw in this case. Is that on-call surgeon just a technician with no relationship with the patient before or after the operation? This view flies in the face of the professional expectations of physicians, who should never abandon their patients [7].

Both shift work and specialization have led to challenges with inter-facility transfers, as we see in this case. Patients are transferred far from home and family support, incurring additional cost, delay in care, and discomfort, in order to receive more specialized care. Often, transfer is appropriate. Determining when a transfer is not appropriate is challenging, but data have revealed that more transfers occur on the weekend [23], and these patients often have worse outcomes [24]. Patient B was transferred to another hospital in the attempt to facilitate specialized and continuous care, but both were ultimately lost. Perhaps he would have been better served receiving care at the first hospital by a qualified general surgeon performing the operation much sooner in his course and then recovering close to home, where his loved ones could frequently visit. In this case, it is possible that a more expedient operation could have resulted in resolution of the obstruction without the need for bowel resection or a second operation, thereby possibly improving Patient B's outcome.

Today's surgeons are bombarded with numerous competing forces and expectations, including but certainly not limited to productivity expectations, outcome metrics, and complicated reimbursement models. All of these and many other factors have led to defensive medicine under the guise of the phrase "I am not comfortable" [25]. Defensive medicine is a complex issue, and the onus is on individual physicians to provide the best care they can provide to each patient entrusted to them, considering primacy for patient welfare and not letting self-interests take precedence, even at the expense of their own convenience and outcome metrics.

Case 2 Ethical Assessment Through a Humanistic Lens

Patient B has undergone a complex and lengthy cancer treatment that has, no doubt, been taxing to him and his family in more ways than one. Throughout this journey, his encounters with his medical team have largely been scheduled electively with the goal of either cure or prolonged survival. His current intervention, while medically not infrequent, is unplanned, as is his sudden decline and rapid death. He and his family may feel abandoned at this critical point at the end of his life, and his own surgeon may also feel a forced distance between herself and her patient. A further wedge may have been driven between the surgeons involved in his care due to local political and financial interests that exacerbated the impersonal nature of Patient B's and his family's experience at this crucial time.

Case 3

Patient C is an 80-year-old retired banker with ovarian cancer that was treated with surgery to remove her uterus, ovaries, and fallopian tubes, followed by chemotherapy and radiation. Recent surveillance imaging revealed liver and lung metastases. She lives alone but has limited mobility, and her daughter visits her once a week to assist with groceries and homemaking. She is currently admitted in the ICU following a massive stroke with poor prospect of functional recovery. It is foreseen that she will not be able to be weaned from the ventilator, so the ICU team has engaged her family members for shared decision-making to discuss possible surgical tracheostomy to allow for long-term mechanical ventilation. The patient's daughter shares that she is distressed to see her mother in such a health state. She recalls her mother telling her many years ago about her wish to never be bedridden in the final days of life and would "rather go" than be a burden to the family. However, the patient's daughter also shares that this is too sudden, and she remains hopeful for a recovery.

The ICU team requests a surgical referral to perform a tracheostomy. The first surgeon assesses her overall condition, particularly in the setting of underlying metastatic cancer, and deems tracheostomy to be non-beneficial care and declines to offer or perform a tracheostomy. The ICU team then consults Dr. S, another surgeon who charges extra fees for referrals that are declined by peers and has always been cooperative by accommodating requests from the ICU team. Dr. S performs the tracheostomy and percutaneous endoscopic gastrostomy tube (PEG) tube placement the next day. Four months later, Patient C is readmitted to the ICU from her long-term acute care (LTAC) facility with septic shock from a urinary tract infection (UTI) in the setting of a chronic indwelling Foley catheter. She has had no neurologic improvement and remains unresponsive and ventilator-dependent. The patient's daughter states that her mother would never have wanted to live the way she had in the LTAC. She expresses regret for agreeing to tracheostomy and PEG, as well as anger at the care team. She desires transition to comfort care, and Patient C passes away peacefully later that evening. The ICU provider asks the Ethics Committee to review her case.

Case 3 Preliminary Ethical Assessment

Patient C is an elderly patient with anticipated devastating neurologic outcome in the setting of underlying metastatic cancer. Tracheostomy would facilitate prolonging a life of functional dependence, which seems to be in opposition to the patient's wishes as stated by her surrogate decision-maker. The first surgeon is justified in declining to offer an operation that is non-beneficial in terms of achieving a desired quality of life. However, because a prognosis is not a guaranteed outcome, it is reasonable to desire a procedure that would allow for prolongation of life in the short-term to allow time for potential neurologic recovery. Therefore, Dr. S was also justified in performing the operation.

7.3.4 Surgeon as a Technician and Loss of Self-regulation

One of the fundamental ethical tenets of medical professionalism is the fiduciary duty to act in the best interests of one's patients, prioritizing their well-being above all else. Most physicians have compassion and service ethos. By hard work, dedication to their craft, and personal sacrifice, they acquire specialized knowledge and technical skills over many years and are legitimately entitled to the fruits of that labor [26]. As physicians earn a living by marketing their knowledge, skills, and experience, their fiduciary duty can conflict with the commercial aspects of healthcare. Physicians, as well as surgeons in particular, can be reduced to technicians whereby they provide services for the patient as a consumer outside of the limits of medical benefit and a traditional physician-patient relationship.

The *1847 AMA Code* also highlighted the professional obligations physicians were to exercise with one another and to the profession at large, including not to "promote oneself in public advertisements, boast of cures, … or hold a patent for an instrument or medication" [7]. These expectations did not persist. While there are valid arguments on all sides of this ethical debate, medicine has become a $4.6 trillion dollar industry in the United States [27], which predictably has raised questions about the ethical boundaries of medical and surgical intervention. Should a medical intervention be offered purely because it is desired by the patient and/or their family? Should a surgeon be a technician and perform tracheostomies and PEG placements for all patients whose families desire them without regard to the prognosis? Should all cosmetic surgery be performed with no limits as long as the patient desires are met? Should the physician's compensation factor into this equation? These questions are complex with no clear answer, but there are ethical limits to what a physician should do or be expected to do. Medical care is much more than a service industry whereby production is determined solely by consumer demand. Rather, physicians have an ethical obligation to their patients to only offer interventions that are expected to benefit, and to not harm, the patients, regardless of demand or financial gain.

A physician's income is generally determined by one of three models: fixed, time-based, or output-based [28]. While fixed and time-based models generally lead to less than appropriate medical care provision, output-based remuneration creates a financial incentive to perform unnecessary procedures by driving physician supplier-induced demand. Fixed income and time-based models disincentivize surgeons, as such models do not adjust for the increased skill requirement and risk accrued in caring for high-risk patients. These models can leave surgeons feeling undervalued and unappreciated with professional frustration and reduced job motivation. It is also possible that financial incentives motivate physicians to provide unnecessary treatment or overcharge patients beyond an "ethical limit" [29]. The concept of reasonableness or the ethical limit for financial gains in medicine is not new. Socrates long ago distinguished between two types of physicians: one motivated by financial gain and the other motivated by a desire to improve patients' lives [30]. He argued that only the latter is a true physician, emphasizing the importance of prioritizing patients' well-being over the temptation of greed. Libertarians argue for a free market in healthcare, emphasizing the importance of liberty in decision-making and pricing. They suggest that as long as transactions are voluntary, any price is justifiable [31]. This perspective allows for charging any amount to a fully informed patient who knowingly chooses a more expensive doctor over cheaper alternatives. Though critical reasoning might justify different pricing in healthcare based on patient purchasing power, expecting doctors to assess each patient's wealth for fair pricing is impractical [32]. To navigate this complexity, regulations and moral guidelines are necessary. Additionally, Gagne and Deci have shown that bringing money into each individual patient interaction erodes the intrinsic physician motivation [33]. While balancing their fiduciary duties with the commercial aspects of healthcare, physicians must maintain their focus on patient welfare as the ultimate factor in their work.

The ethical requirement to prioritize patient welfare does not mean that the physician's personal needs are eclipsed. There are now more parties involved in the interaction, which may feel like more of a transaction. Because healthcare in the United States is still not considered to be a basic human right for all, most healthcare systems are built on the model of for-profit industries, with their attendant motivations and threats. In for-profit models, there may be pressure to prioritize financial considerations over patient care, potentially leading to practices that prioritize profit-making procedures. Despite attempted protections in the setting of medical emergencies, the presence or absence of health insurance dictates the type of care that can be provided along the course of the disease and treatment. But it has also led to the entry of another party in the social contract—the payor. Because patients are rarely self-pay, as very few could afford current healthcare costs alone, the payor almost always enters the equation. While in other markets, the buyer helps to set the price with demand, the same cannot be done in medicine, as it is much more challenging to set a price on health and functionality. Instead, government entities and insurance companies have set prices and payments, thereby introducing a new party of potentially "unqualified practitioners" [4] into the contract and the erosion of the influence of physicians on the delivery of healthcare to society.

The introduction of new parties into the physician-patient relationship has contributed to erosion of trust beyond the financial concerns already discussed. Well-intended organizational systems aimed at improving patient safety, such as outcome reporting databases, carry hidden incentives that favor low-risk and socioeconomically advantaged patients with good health insurance. Salary and bonus structures reward expensive and sometimes unnecessary procedures. Laws regulating what and how medical care can be delivered to patients have often been made by non-clinicians, thereby prohibiting physicians from delivering the care they believe is indicated and is in their patients' best interests. Perhaps most importantly, these factors contribute significantly to health disparities, adverse medical outcomes, and physician and provider burnout. Physicians must ensure that they are included in the social dialogue and policy-making to ensure that laws surrounding the practice of medicine are both scientifically and ethically appropriate.

The privilege of self-regulation in the medical profession includes the responsibility, authority, and absolute obligation to promulgate impeccable standards of education, training, and practice to guarantee the competence of members for upholding the primary commitment to serve the public good [34, 35]. Once a trustworthy moral enterprise, the medical profession is now increasingly perceived as prioritizing self-interests and shielding the incompetent under the guise of collegiality, with heightened skepticism that the profession has failed to self-regulate [36]. McAneny et al. suggest three domains that could be addressed to enhance effectiveness of self-regulation: i.e., addressing individual physician misconduct, integrating strong professionalism in medical education, and managing organizational and care delivery practices that may compromise professionalism among practicing physicians [37]. Ensuring accountability for lapses in professional conduct is essential for self-regulation. This task requires improved understanding of risk factors, effective intervention strategies, and fair mechanisms to identify and address unsafe practices. Political interference in the form of government and insurance industry regulations can impact medical decision-making and self-regulation. Thus, self-regulation should constructively interface with local sociopolitical and cultural norms [38]. The AMA is dedicated to improving self-regulation in medicine by strengthening oversight, supporting state medical boards, educating physicians on professionalism, and addressing practice stressors to prevent misconduct and uphold professional standards [10].

Case 3 Ethical Assessment Through a Humanistic Lens
Performing a tracheostomy on Patient C would allow for life prolongation as well as facilitate discharge from the hospital to an LTAC facility. Both offering and declining to offer tracheostomy can be appropriate, depending upon the wishes of the patient. Because those are unknown, the surgeon must rely on shared decision-making with the patient's daughter, and this decision-making model requires weighing benefits and burdens of interventions. It is not clear that Dr. S weighed these considerations. Financial benefit to the surgeon should never outweigh what is best for the patient.

7.4 The Modern-Day "Contract"

The social contract has never been an explicit binding document. The earliest written form, over 150 years ago, included numerous expectations that would today be considered out of date, if not outright foolish (e.g., patients not seeking "second opinions," the expectation for patients to unquestionably obey physicians' orders, etc.) [7]. Numerous published revisions have been made between 1903 and 2016 that focus more on professional obligations of physicians rather than on mutual expectations between multiple parties [7, 9].

The social contract has evolved over time in response to changes within the field of medicine and throughout society. The medical profession must continuously adapt to these changes while also maintaining the core tenets of the contract in order to maintain both the integrity of the profession and society's trust. We have already experienced the consequences of poor individual behavior, widespread misinformation, escalating healthcare costs, and lack of transparency. These consequences—which are too numerous to name and involve countless victims—have weakened the reciprocal nature of the contract, including what physicians expect in return for their work and sacrifices (i.e., autonomy, status, rewards, and monopoly). A resultant disillusionment has exacerbated physician burnout [39].

In a rapidly changing healthcare milieu, there are seemingly endless ethical issues to discuss and debate. Loss of trust, health disparities, increased specialization, shift work, the surgeon as a merchant, and loss of self-regulation are far from a comprehensive list of the ethical concerns of surgeons today, but they do effectively frame our discussion of our role and responsibility to our patients and society as a whole (i.e., our place in the social contract). As physicians, our place has always centered on the responsibility to uphold the contract by maintaining high professional standards. We have been the bearers of trust. New parties have been added to the contract—including hospital systems, policy-makers, and third-party payors—but they have not been bound by the same fiduciary requirements as physicians have. Instead, their powers are linked to finances and have thus been perceived as untrustworthy [11]. Yet, their powers are significant over both patients and physicians. As a result, physicians have found themselves in an often-precarious position—one where their obligations to the patient are in opposition to that of the larger system or payor, where the ability to appropriately or equitably care for the patient is limited by those parties. Physicians understand this conflict, but patients often do not. Therefore, physicians should have more decision-making responsibility regarding policy, resource allocation, coverage, and reimbursement. In exchange, they must uphold the social contract by being transparent about their own interests and motivations.

The addition of a humanistic lens to our ethical evaluations of individual cases, particularly the ethically challenging ones, can aid in ensuring that the patient's unique perspective, experiences, and beliefs are considered. This consideration will improve our understanding of the patient overall, strengthen the physician-patient relationship, and potentially improve our decision-making.

References

1. Definition of humanism [Internet]. American Humanist Association. [cited 2024 May 7]. Available from: https://americanhumanist.org/what-is-humanism/definition-of-humanism/#:~:text=Humanism%20is%20an%20approach%20to,and%20life%20in%20a%20hereafter
2. Stevenson A. Oxford dictionary of English [Internet]. Oxford University Press; 2010. Available from: https://www.oxfordreference.com/view/10.1093/acref/9780199571123.001.0001/acref-9780199571123

3. Indla V, Radhika MS. Hippocratic oath: losing relevance in today's world? Indian J Psychiatry. 2019;61(Suppl 4):S773–5.
4. Wynia MK. The short history and tenuous future of medical professionalism: the erosion of Medicine's social contract. Perspect Biol Med. 2008;51(4):565–78.
5. Noda CH, Brown D, Kopar PK. The surgeon as a professional: changes and challenges over time. Ann Surg. 2023;278(2):179–83.
6. Professionalism and medicine's social contract with society. AMA J Ethics [Internet]. 2004 [cited 2023 Feb 8];6(4). Available from: https://journalofethics.ama-assn.org/article/professionalism-and-medicines-social-contract-society/2004-04
7. Isaac H, Francis Condie D, Emerson G, Fox G, Bridges R, Norris GW, Morris C, West F, Paul JR. The code of medical ethics of the American Medical Association [Internet]. T. K. And P. G. Collins, Printers; 1847. Available from: https://www.ama-assn.org/sites/ama-assn.org/files/corp/media-browser/public/ethics/1847code_0.pdf
8. Cruess SR, Cruess RL. Professionalism and medicine's social contract with society. AMA J Ethics [Internet]. 2004 Apr 1 [cited 2023 Aug 29];6(4). Available from: https://journalofethics.ama-assn.org/article/professionalism-and-medicines-social-contract-society/2004-04
9. History of the code [internet]. American Medical Association; 2017. Available from: https://www.ama-assn.org/sites/ama-assn.org/files/corp/media-browser/public/ethics/ama-code-ethics-history.pdf
10. Brotherton S, Kao A, Crigger BJ. Professing the values of medicine: the modernized AMA code of medical ethics. JAMA. 2016;316(10):1041–2.
11. Blendon RJ, Benson JM. Trust in Medicine, the Health System & Public Health. Daedalus. 2022;151(4):67–82.
12. Working Party of the Royal College of Physicians. Doctors in society. Medical professionalism in a changing world. Clin Med (Lond). 2005;5(6 Suppl 1):S5–40.
13. Resneck J Jr. Turning the tide against medical disinformation will take all of us [Internet]. American Medical Association; 2022. [cited 2024 Mar 27]. Available from: https://www.ama--assn.org/about/leadership/turning-tide-against-medical-disinformation-will-take-all-us
14. Read DJ, Bradbury R, Yeboah E. Firework-related injury in the top end: a 16-year review. ANZ J Surg. 2017;87(12):1030–4.
15. Read L, Nelson H, Korenda L. Rebuilding trust in health care. Deloitte Insights. 2021 Aug 5
16. Baciu A, Negussie Y, Geller A, et al. The state of health disparities in the United States. In: Communities in action: pathways to health equity [internet]. National Academies Press; 2017. Available from: https://www-ncbi-nlm-nih-gov.beckerproxy.wustl.edu/books/NBK425844/.
17. Dean W, Talbot S, Dean A. Reframing clinician distress: moral injury not burnout. Fed Pract. 2019;36(9):400–2.
18. Marks AR. Doctors from hell: the horrific account of Nazi experiments on humans. J Clin Invest. 2006;116(1):2.
19. Robeznieks A. Legacy of racial segregation endures at many U.S. hospitals [internet]. AMA. 2021. Available from: https://www.ama-assn.org/delivering-care/health-equity/legacy-racial-segregation-endures-many-us-hospitals
20. Chapman EN, Kaatz A, Carnes M. Physicians and implicit bias: how doctors may unwittingly perpetuate health care disparities. J Gen Intern Med. 2013;28(11):1504–10.
21. Levy-Carrick NC, Lewis-O'Connor A, Rittenberg E, Manosalvas K, Stoklosa HM, Silbersweig DA. Promoting health equity through trauma-informed care: critical role for physicians in policy and program development. Fam Community Health. 2019;42(2):104–8.
22. SAMHSA's concept of trauma and guidance for a trauma-informed approach [internet]. Department of Health & Human Services; 2014. Available from: https://nicic.gov/samhsas-concept-trauma-and-guidance-trauma-informed-approach
23. Moore A, Waxman MJ, Reid S, Wu A, Ata A, Telisky A, et al. Trends in interfacility transfer volume by season, day of week, time of day, and federal holiday status. JEM Rep. 2023;2(2):100026.

24. Mueller SK, Fiskio J, Schnipper J. Interhospital transfer: transfer processes and patient outcomes. J Hosp Med. 2019;14(8):486–91.
25. Jurkovich GJ. I am not comfortable with this: 2020 scudder oration on trauma. J Am Coll Surg. 2021;232(3):231–40.
26. Jones JW, McCullough LB, Richman BW. Show me the money: the ethics of physicians' income. J Vasc Surg. 2005;42(2):377–9.
27. National health expenditure data [Internet]. CMSgov 2023. Available from: https://www.cms.gov/data-research/statistics-trends-and-reports/national-health-expenditure-data/historical#:~:text=U.S.%20health%20care%20spending%20grew,trillion%20or%20%2413%2C493%20per%20person
28. Woodward RS, Warren-Boulton F. Considering the effects of financial incentives and professional ethics on 'appropriate' medical care. J Health Econ. 1984;3(3):223–37.
29. Eric H. When doctors overcharge, what price do they pay? [Internet]. Singapore L Rev Available from: https://www.singaporelawreview.com/juris-illuminae-entries/2015/when-doctors-overcharge-what-price-do-they-pay
30. Gunderman RB, Hubbard MA. The wages of healing: ethical issues in the compensation of physicians. Med Sci Monit. 2005;11(2):SR5–10.
31. Wong G, Tan L, Yap P. A moral price for medicine. SMEDJ. 2015;56(07):363–5.
32. Singer P. Practical ethics [Internet]. 3rd ed. Cambridge University Press; 2011. Available from: https://assets.cambridge.org/97805218/81418/frontmatter/9780521881418_frontmatter.pdf
33. Gagné M, Deci EL. Self-determination theory and work motivation. J Organ Behav. 2005;26(4):331–62.
34. Cardenas CJ. Self-regulation of the medical profession and maintenance of certification. JAMA. 2018;319(1):83.
35. Cruess SR, Johnston S, Cruess RL. Professionalism for medicine: opportunities and obligations. Iowa Orthop J. 2004;24:9–14.
36. The medical profession and self-regulation: a current challenge. AMA J Ethics [Internet] 2005 Apr 1 [cited 2024 May 2];7(4). Available from: https://journalofethics.ama-assn.org/article/medical-profession-and-self-regulation-current-challenge/2005-04
37. McAneny BL, Crigger EJ. Toward more effective self-regulation in medicine. Am J Bioeth. 2019;19(1):7–10.
38. Mansoori A, Schantz E. ICoME and the legitimacy of professional self-regulation. J Med Ethics. 2023;50:jme-2023.
39. Rothstein A. Physician burnout. National Affairs. 2024, Winter.

Chapter 8
Preoperative Evaluation and Discussion: Trust as the Foundation

Andrew J. Neevel and Norman D. Hogikyan

8.1 Introduction

Ms. M had seen multiple physicians over the years and heard many possible explanations for her worsening breathing difficulty. Asthma, although not supported by objective testing, was considered the top possibility, yet trials of asthma treatment were never effective [1, 2]. As she settled into the possibility that this was simply her normal condition, her breathing became noisier with a high-pitched sound when inhaling, prompting referral to an otolaryngologist—an ear, nose, and throat physician. She was skeptical as to why she was seeing yet another physician in a field she did not think of as being related to breathing problems but followed through with the recommendation. Three months later, she was sitting in an exam room awaiting a physician whom she had not previously met, but she was comforted by knowing he did have good online reviews and was affiliated with a reputable medical center.

The doctor entered the exam room, learned about her history of breathing problems, numbed her throat with a bitter-tasting spray, performed an examination with a flexible endoscope, and said that he now understood the cause of her breathing problems. She was informed that she had a narrowing in her airway called subglottic stenosis and that she was breathing through an opening reduced to less than half

A. J. Neevel
Department of Otolaryngology-Head & Neck Surgery, University of Michigan, Ann Arbor, MI, USA
e-mail: ajneevel@med.umich.edu

N. D. Hogikyan (✉)
Department of Otolaryngology-Head & Neck Surgery, University of Michigan, Ann Arbor, MI, USA

University of Michigan Center for Bioethics and Social Sciences in Medicine, Ann Arbor, MI, USA
e-mail: nhogikya@med.umich.edu

F. Jotterand, C. Bosco (eds.), *Fostering Humanism in Surgery*, New Paradigms in Healthcare, https://doi.org/10.1007/978-3-031-82771-6_8

of what it should be. The doctor recommended further testing to determine the cause of the problem, while acknowledging that it is often idiopathic (i.e., unknown). Surgery was recommended to widen the airway to improve her breathing, and the doctor reviewed the reasons for this recommendation, as well as the associated surgical risks and potential benefits. Ms. M had never heard of breathing problems requiring surgical treatment, and was initially a bit overwhelmed by the examination, diagnosis, and discussion of surgery. She did not anticipate any of this prior to the office visit and was both frightened yet grateful for a diagnosis and proposed treatment plan.

Based on your own experiences, how might you feel in this patient's position? How would you respond to these new faces, unexpected information, and decisions to be made? What if your breathing worsened dramatically and you presented to the emergency room instead of the outpatient clinic? What dynamics in the case would make you more or less comfortable with the surgical plan? And ultimately, what would result in trusting this surgeon with not just your breathing problem but potentially your life?

The public perception and media portrayal of surgical practice tends to emphasize technical skill in the operating room, yet surgeons themselves recognize that decision-making and the individualization of patient care planning are often the most challenging and critical parts of their profession. The steps of a surgical procedure can be repeated over and over until mastered, while questions pertaining to whether and/or when to proceed with surgery for a particular patient can be much more nuanced. These questions should incorporate not only the patient's clinical circumstances but also their values, goals, and preferences. Core bioethical principles of beneficence, nonmaleficence, respect for autonomy, and justice inform decision-making, while real-world shared decision-making comes down to determining what is right and good for a particular patient in a particular situation [3, 4].

This thoughtful individualization of patient care is in many ways an expression of humanism in medicine or humanistic clinical practice. While definitions of humanism in the medical context will vary, a fundamental goal can be stated as the prioritization of patient welfare and encouragement of human flourishing. Key components of medical humanism have been described as the 3C's: comprehension, compassion, and commitment [5]. Physician attitudes and behaviors that engender humanism in the clinical setting include whole-person care, valuing, perspective-taking, relational focus, and recognizing universality [6]. Establishing a human-to-human connection between surgeon and patient is a valuable foundation for important decision-making that will take place along the care pathway.

Much of this decision-making occurs in an initial clinical encounter in the outpatient office setting, or, less commonly, when seen in the emergency department or admitted to the hospital for more acute problems. A patient may present with a previously undiagnosed constellation of symptoms and neither they nor the surgeon initially know that surgery will be the recommended treatment. In other cases, the patient may present with a clear prior diagnosis whereby surgery is the anticipated treatment plan. In a relatively short period of time, the surgeon will introduce themselves, review available records, complete a thorough history and physical examination, formulate a diagnosis and treatment plan, educate, and then counsel the patient.

From the patient's perspective, they will meet a new physician, discuss personal and sometimes intimate details of their life, undergo physical examination, and then must both assimilate and assess their circumstance. The preoperative evaluation must include discussion of risks and benefits of recommended treatments and potential alternative treatments. Discussion, questions, and answers typically follow and culminate in a shared treatment decision. This process constitutes informed consent for surgery, which is then typically acknowledged by signing a consent form. It is the discussion of the surgeon and the patient that is important; the signing of the consent simply codifies the discussion.

Now while the preceding discussion denotes the details of a preoperative visit, there is so much more than information exchange occurring during this seemingly straightforward clinical encounter. While the transactional elements of the relationship are readily visible, the relational elements are less apparent and, arguably, more consequential. The physician is duty-bound to have the patient's best interest in mind, and yet assuring the patient of their shared humanistic goals can pose another layer of challenges. Patients may speak with their surgeon very little on the actual day of surgery, and therefore this initial clinical encounter may be one of the only opportunities to establish the dyadic and essential surgeon-patient relationship. We propose that trust is foundational to preoperative evaluation and the relationship experienced by both surgeon and patient. In this chapter we will explore the development of trust during the preoperative evaluation, reflect upon its significance, and explore how contemporary medicine and surgery can both engender and challenge the establishment and maintenance of this trust.

8.2 Defining Trust

Trust. You may "know it when you feel it," but exactly what is it? The fundamental meaning of trust is understood intuitively, and yet it is a multidimensional concept with specifics that are dependent upon the context. We place trust in institutions, groups, individuals, and ourselves [7, 8]. Prior experience greatly informs trust, while additional experiences can build or break a previously established trust. A distilled definition of trust is the optimistic acceptance of vulnerability wherein the trustor believes the trustee will care for their interests [9].

Optimism, in this context, requires a belief that a trusting relationship can be fruitful. It corresponds with the underlying hope that the trustee, be it an individual or institution, is trustworthy [10]. Trustworthiness is a property related to trust, though fundamentally different. Trust is an attitude or belief in another party's trustworthiness [11]. Different parties may be inherently more willing to trust despite less perceived trustworthiness, depending upon their personal judgment. An individual with greater optimism or hope may be more likely to accept vulnerability in a trusting relationship. Greater vulnerability, like a patient with a rare disease or acutely worsening symptoms, also may compel an individual to trust their doctor, as their optimism is related to survival or desperation, not necessarily perceived trustworthiness.

Vulnerability can include both parties with a different power dynamic, as long as both are fully invested in the results. For example, a patient trusts their doctor to provide accurate medical advice, and a doctor prescribes a course of treatment that includes a close monitoring plan because they trust the patient to return for follow-up. The patient is a vulnerable party in both scenarios, and the doctor's investment in that patient's well-being also makes them vulnerable. In either case, both parties are, or should be, committed to the best interest of the patient. Despite the surgeon's own determination of a patient's trustworthiness, the surgeon has a professional responsibility to enter a trust-based relationship [12]. This is simply stated in the first chapter of the American Medical Association's Code of Ethics: "The relationship between a patient and a physician is based on trust, which gives rise to physicians' ethical responsibility to place patients' welfare above the physician's own self-interest" [13]. Furthermore, the American College of Surgeons (ACS) Code of Professional Conduct states: "As Fellows of the American College of Surgeons, we treasure the trust that our patients have placed in us because trust is integral to the practice of surgery" [14].

Predicated on the significant imbalance in vulnerability, the physician holds the greater responsibility compared to that of the patient. The ACS Code of Professional Conduct states that the responsibilities of a surgeon include the requirement to: "Be sensitive and respectful of patients, understanding their vulnerability during the perioperative period" [14]. The AMA Code of Ethics additionally states, "physicians must also uphold ethical responsibilities not to discriminate against a prospective patient on the basis of race, gender, sexual orientation or gender identity, or other personal or social characteristics that are not clinically relevant to the individual's care. Nor may physicians decline a patient based solely on the individual's infectious disease status" [13].

The physician has a professional responsibility to foster trust with the patient, but there are circumstances in which the patient breaks the physician's trust in them. This could be an inability to follow through with a treatment plan, lack of expected follow-up, or a patient's behavioral challenges. Important to this discussion is the caveat that these challenges may be secondary to social determinants of health, health literacy, or health inequities [15, 16]. Socioeconomic factors beyond a patient's control can impact such things as their ability to obtain prescribed medications, follow nutritional or wound care guidelines, or present for postoperative care at a designated time or place. A patient may have preconceived beliefs or opinions about doctors or the healthcare system that are rooted in personal lived experience or a historical perspective, and these can challenge the establishment and maintenance of trust with a new physician. Often, thoughtful inquiry, discussion, and openness to learning and understanding can bridge a gap between patient and physician, and also define steps to mitigate negative effects of particular contextual features. Ideally, this inquiry and learning process is bidirectional, and yet the greatest responsibility in this regard will always rest with the surgeon.

The concept of "therapeutic trust" is an interesting, though potentially paternalistic, concept. Therapeutic trust would be when, despite the doctor's assessment of lower trustworthiness in the patient, they will offer an opportunity to follow through and build trust [12]. Carter further introduces the concept of "overriding" therapeutic trust, in which a successful opportunity to trust both achieves the present goal and builds trust between parties [17]. For example, patients electing to undergo bariatric surgery are often required to participate in rigorous diet and exercise programs before proceeding. Successful participation directly improves the outcomes of surgery, but also reassures the surgeon that the patient can conform to difficult postoperative restrictions. Even in more unidirectional surgical relationships, when the patient is most vulnerable, surgeons must trust their patient to complete preoperative expectations, report accurate symptoms, and follow through with required postoperative care.

In morbid operations that require long hospital stays, a surgeon performs a case and provides the opportunity and support for a patient to be restored to an increased measure of health. Surgeons hold high expectations for this surgical "buy-in" of a patient on whom they decide to operate, describing the entire process as a "package deal" [18]. In untrustworthy patients, a surgeon may decide to employ therapeutic trust and perform the surgery anyway with an acceptance of the risk that their outcomes might be compromised by patient adherence to the recommended plan. However, if this idea is employed by the surgeon, it must be carefully weighed with the risks and benefits of the procedure and the patient's preference as determined through the lens of shared decision-making. This is easier said than done. Surgeons notably struggle with defaulting to paternalism when patients do not follow through postoperatively, and many experienced surgeons do recognize the concept of benevolent paternalism as a patient-centered practice [19]. If the patient who met preoperative bariatric surgery expectations decided that they wanted to eat on their first day after surgery, which would risk significant harm at the surgical site, the surgeon and hospital staff would tell them that the caregivers knew better, likely provide graphic descriptions of the negative consequences of eating at that time, and not provide food to the patient. Surgeons generally assume that a patient will accept life-saving treatment if postoperative complications arise, yet qualitative work has shown that patients expect to have some limitations to interventions not discussed preoperatively [20]. Next, we will examine how trust is established in the preoperative evaluation.

8.3 Preoperative Evaluation and Trust

The preoperative evaluation is a key and potentially the only opportunity to establish trust in the surgeon-patient relationship prior to surgery. As described in our case example or more commonly in an emergency, in a short period of time, a surgeon and patient may discuss a serious symptom and diagnosis and enter into a highly consequential professional contract. Many times, this unique interaction begins with no prior direct relationship and culminates with an agreement by an individual to entrust their well-being and potentially their life into the hands of another person.

Prior to a patient stepping into an exam room and personally meeting a surgeon, a variety of influences are at play. Larger historical, social, and media influences and context may affect a patient's anticipation of a surgeon they have yet to meet. Access itself was found to be an influencing factor in the development of trust in a cohort of patients with less healthcare interactions per year [21]. Individual past experiences also impact a patient's state of mind and, to some degree, their willingness to trust their surgeon. Although clearly secondary to the direct interpersonal connection formed during the clinical encounter, the influence of these feelings prior to the actual preoperative visit was identified as a theme in qualitative research by Hogikyan et al. into how trust develops in the surgeon-patient relationship [22]. Patients cited their own personal experiences with doctors, online reviews, and institutional reputation as notable factors in their willingness to trust. In other literature, however, time spent researching symptoms and physician profiles did not correlate with perceived patient trust in hand surgeons, which supports the importance of their in-person impressions of their surgeon [23].

No doubt an individual would rather undergo surgery by a surgeon whom they trust as opposed to one for whom they have not had the opportunity to develop trust, or one they may distrust. While patients undoubtedly value the technical skills of a surgeon and desire the best outcomes, they routinely identify personal connections as central to their trust in a surgeon. A qualitative study on effective ways that surgeons establish trust in patients with pancreatic cancer found that optimistic honesty, approachability, good communication, appreciating patient values, and family member input were most impactful [24]. Similarly, patients identified fidelity, competence, and honesty as engendering trust in their oncologists [25]. Another study found technical ability, verbal communication skills, and respect for a patient's autonomy to be most important in hand surgeons [26]. And finally, our own qualitative study referenced above utilizing thematic analysis of patient interviews regarding trust development in the surgeon-patient relationship found that interpersonal connection developed during the clinical encounter was the most important factor in the development of trust [22]. Similar to other studies, such things as kindness, honesty, and good communication skills were highlighted by patients. How a surgeon was observed communicating and interacting with other members of their clinical team was also noted as a factor in trust development, and, as discussed later in this chapter, this has important implications for how preoperative surgical evaluation care is coordinated.

The approach of shared decision-making is critical to the early development of trust, demonstrated in both qualitative and quantitative measures of trust [27, 28]. Shared decision-making is a process of communicating risk, clarifying patient values, and jointly arriving at a decision [29–31]. Not only can this approach align outcomes with patient values, but the process of incorporating goals and preferences increases patient trust in their surgeon [32]. Humility and transparency also reassure patients, which can lead to better health utilization. Well-established trust and a direct recognition of uncertainty can decrease unnecessary tests and overtreatment [33]. Patients feel a greater sense of safety during their hospital stay when trust is established with their surgeon [34]. Patients also appreciate when surgeons disclosed their specialty bias or offered consultation with another specialist [35].

A critical juncture of the preoperative consultation is obtaining informed consent. The informed consent process has three cornerstones: preconditions (competence, willingness), information (diagnosis, prognosis, risks, benefits, alternatives), and legal consent [36]. The patient must demonstrate that they have capacity, which requires the ability to understand the necessary information, appreciate the significance of the situation, reason through the decision, and communicate a choice [37, 38]. This is necessary to ensure the patient's autonomy is preserved when agreeing to medical treatment [39].

Patients expect and are entitled to more than these check boxes. Surveyed patients from New Zealand were asked to select "important" and, separately, "preferred" information in the preoperative setting. The most important topics were options for treatment, common risks, meeting the surgeon, and the technique used. Preferred items were recovery time, options for treatment, legal rights, and again, meeting the surgeon [40]. Meeting the surgeon was identified as both important and preferred by patients, suggesting that patients perceive their relationship with their surgeon as a required element of the informed consent process and personally valuable. This illustrates how critical the early surgeon-patient relationship, and the ensuing foundation for trust, is to patients in the informed consent process.

While the basic framework for informed consent is helpful in medicolegal discussion, the true attainment of "informed" prior to consent is intensely subjective and variable when considering health literacy, patient preference, previous knowledge, and significance of risks. Informed consent for a complex cardiothoracic procedure should be held to the same ethical standard as a laceration repair, but achieving informed consent requires significantly more effort by both the surgeon and patient. Nonetheless, a graphic description of a sternotomy ("cracking open your chest") may be unnecessarily frightening for the patient. Even the most experienced patient counselor will never replace years of surgical education and training. Gabay et al. performed a narrative study to provide the basis for an informed consent process model that incorporates patient autonomy into information disclosure [41]. While the core components of informed consent are necessary, additional discussion should be tailored to "patient needs, emotional state, and preferences." Practical ways to consider patient preference for information include asking "how do you like to receive medical information – every detail or an overall summary?" Even without perfect understanding, the patient's autonomy and moral agency are better preserved throughout the entire consent process when their preferences are considered from the start.

Patients may mistrust their surgeons or hold reservations based on preconceptions or personal experience. This poses a unique challenge for surgeons meeting a patient for the first time, as the patient may have less optimism regarding the surgeon's interest in their well-being. Sullivan presents the idea that medical professionals often respond to an "atmosphere of mistrust" by stressing their competence and caring, matching our fundamental definition of trust [42]. Yet, without the patient's optimism or willingness, these attempts are potentially inconsequential. Rather, Sullivan suggests that taking the risk to recognize existing mistrust is an important step in demonstrating trustworthiness. Education and awareness are crucial for being able to engage in sensitive conversations with patients of different backgrounds [43].

Risk-taking in acknowledging barriers to trust applies to more than existing mistrust. Recognition of a patient's underlying emotions or reactions to their clinical environment or information given to them is critical. If these barriers are not understood and discussed by the surgeon, they may limit building trust initially and may jeopardize continued trust. Communication strategies like asking open-ended questions and voicing observations (e.g. "my mention of the possibility of cancer seemed to really worry you") and thoughtful, active listening can provide a patient the opportunity to describe their concerns up front. Not only can recognition of these factors improve the surgeon-patient relationship, but it can also guide discussion and choices during shared decision-making. Indeed, meeting a patient "where they live" and speaking human being-to-human being are immensely valuable for both parties on the road to surgeon-patient trust.

Surgeon and institutional reputation may have additional implications when patients consider the larger picture of their surgical care. Langerman et al. studied patient perceptions of overlapping surgery, where the attending surgeon, whom they met during their preoperative evaluation oversees two cases at once with less-experienced fellows and residents performing intermittently unsupervised surgery [44]. The fact that many patients were comfortable with this prospect exhibits the power of institutional and professional reputation. Past negative experiences were found to have an impact on patients' comfort with overlapping surgery, which illustrates how they perceive the institution, supervision, and trainees. Patient perception of the individual surgeon and the institution are reciprocal and influence one another over time [9].

At the end, in a postoperative visit following surgery, the patient finally has comprehensive information to inform their trust in their surgeon. They experienced the surgeon's expertise, bedside manner, and the entire process of surgery. Some surgeon-patient relationships end at this point, while others continue. This can be the case in routine postoperative follow-up, chronic diseases, or complications. Interestingly, patients' continued trust is not necessarily outcome-related. A strong relationship with open communication maintained patient trust in colorectal surgery patients who experienced complications [45]. This suggests that communication, relationship-building, and early management of expectations are critical for maintaining a trusting surgeon-patient relationship that can supersede negative outcomes.

8.4 The Trust Crisis and Modern Obstacles

Recent publications in the Harvard Business Review and Massachusetts General Hospital magazine have discussed a modern trust crisis in the business and corporate world, and in medicine, with changes in stakeholder relationships at the core of the crises [46, 47]. The surgeon-patient relationship, one of the most consequential relationships in medicine and arguably in society at large, is not immune to contemporary challenges for the development of trust. At the turn of this century, Axelrod and Goold published an insightful paper on how to maintain trust in the surgeon-patient relationship in the new millennium [48]. They expressed concerns about potential threats to maintaining trust including surgeons prioritizing technical prowess over meaningful relationships; the shift toward outpatient procedures decreasing patient and surgeon contact time while adding to family member care burden; sensationalized publicizing of greed, fraud, and abuse in the medical community; and the perception of exploitation by an economically successful medical industry. They posited that improvements can be made by visible surgeon advocacy for the health and economic well-being of their patients, investment in surgical trainee psychosocial development, higher credentialing and oversight policies, and patient outcomes research.

Some of these concerns have been addressed in the past two decades, with clear opportunity for further improvement. Biopsychosocial learning has been integrated into requirements from premedical undergraduate curricula to the professional development of attending physicians. Medical schools and residencies now select applicants based on criteria that include communication skills, empathy, and readiness to work in teams. Advocacy has become further solidified as part of a physician's identity. Nonetheless, in just two years of the COVID-19 pandemic, trust in physicians plummeted from 40% to 29% according to Pew Research [49]. A new set of modern challenges for surgeon-patient trust development have arisen. Many are too broad and complex to discuss here; therefore, in the following section, we will focus on several specific areas that may impact trust formation in the preoperative evaluation. These include administrative and electronic documentation burdens, virtual care, physician burnout, staffing model changes, and corporate healthcare ownership. We believe that anything that alters how surgeons interact with their patients can introduce concessions that have the potential to undermine trust. It is essential to the future of our profession that we are mindful of this possibility and faithfully work to mitigate it.

8.4.1 Administrative and Electronic Documentation Burdens

The growing physician administrative and electronic documentation burdens associated with contemporary healthcare delivery detract from meaningful time spent with patients and also contribute to physician burnout [50, 51]. Physicians and patients each recognize that time invested in cultivating the doctor-patient relationship is key to establishing trust. Yet other demands that are patient care-adjacent can reduce this time in more and more invasive ways. What patient, or physician, has not lamented the amount of time spent looking at a screen or typing on a keyboard rather than focused, personal attention on the developing dyadic relationship? There are a myriad of other less visible actions as well that are associated with care delivery in complex modern healthcare systems, and even a seemingly straightforward step such as ordering a diagnostic study, prescribing a medication, or scheduling a procedure can trigger a series of authorization, justification, certification, denial, and appeal tasks. While other medical and administrative team members can perform some of these tasks, many ultimately fall to the physician, thus further compromising time for more direct patient-facing activities. While some of these changes may improve objective measures of efficiency and cost-effective healthcare delivery, they come at the expense of interpersonal interaction that has great value, though is more difficult to assess. Maintaining the human element is critical for both surgeon and patient, as satisfaction for both is tied to their interactions.

8.4.2 Virtual Care Models

A rapid adoption of virtual care occurred by necessity during the COVID-19 pandemic and was a forced experiment with this model [52]. Recognizing that this represented an abrupt, even seismic, shift in the doctor-patient relationship, Hogikyan and Shuman, each clinical ethicists and otolaryngologists, explored how the pandemic impacted otolaryngologists and their doctor-patient relationships [53]. Observations included: "The road that we currently travel must include trust and trustworthiness as a destination, and communication is unquestionably our primary vehicle. Established patients will need to understand why symptoms that previously warranted direct hands-on care are now being approached remotely." and, "At a time when even simple human contact is a risk factor for disease, we argue that a human "touch"—be it virtual, verbal, or otherwise—remains a vital part of care".

For primary care patients, one study found that virtual care satisfactorily established trust, even in the absence of an initial in-person meeting occurred [54]. However, in a group of Black adults receiving oncology care, virtual care offered a perceived lack of interpersonal connectedness [55]. There is a paucity of research specific to surgery regarding the establishment of trust in virtual care models. As surgeons, our personal experience finds virtual care is best-suited to be incorporated into previously established surgeon-patient relationships and for routine follow-up post-procedure regarding easily reportable symptoms or signs. Additionally, it is logical that the gravity and nature of the care offered should guide the appropriateness of virtual care. A study found that for a patient undergoing a hernia repair, a virtual preoperative assessment had similar satisfaction levels but with cost savings compared to in-person care [56]. Katta et al. suggest that appropriate use of virtual care may actually build trust in surgical care, by extending access, using technology to improve literacy-adjusted education, and meeting a patient in the comfort of their home [57]. In the post-pandemic world, we can be more thoughtful about where to incorporate the virtual care model. Maintaining choice for both patient and surgeon is integral to preserving, or establishing, a trusting relationship. Variation in comfort level with virtual care may shift over time at a population level, yet this should not replace individual surgeons and patients discussing whether or how to incorporate virtual care into a particular surgeon-patient relationship.

8.4.3 Surgeon of the Day and Handoffs for Elective Care

It is typical for on-call responsibilities to be shared by surgeons within a particular group practice on a schedule determined by institutional norms. Clinical encounters while on-call may include new or established patients with urgent or emergent problems, and both surgeons and patients recognize that the availability of care is generally prioritized over patient choice to see a particular doctor even if they are an established patient. While some surgeons and circumstances will still facilitate treatment by their surgeon for established patients, a patient's expectation for a preexisting preoperative relationship rightfully changes in an emergency setting.

In some elective situations, however, a related model is utilized. A patient may undergo a preoperative evaluation by one surgeon, yet, depending upon the timing of their scheduled operation, they may be operated on by a different surgeon. Logistically, this arrangement can improve efficiency and timeliness for both patients and surgical practices. Wait times no longer correspond to individual surgeon availability; rather, they are averaged across the practice. Advanced practice providers (physician assistants and nurse practitioners) can also fit into this model by routinely performing preoperative evaluations and postoperative assessments. In this instance, the patients do not necessarily meet their surgeon before the day of surgery. This allows more operative days for the surgeon, which, in many cases, is their primary revenue-generating activity.

While this model may enhance scheduling efficiency and potentially revenue generation, we ask at what cost to the trust issues we have discussed? The lack of continuity presents a host of challenges that have the potential to erode trust, or to simply prevent it from being established initially. Separating the roles of patient evaluation and counseling from performance of the actual surgical procedure diminishes the surgeon-patient relationship and can promote the perception that being a surgeon is purely a technical exercise. The fallacy of this notion is obvious to established surgeons. We believe it is vital to the future of the profession that those physicians who practice and teach surgical disciplines not only take a holistic approach to surgical care themselves but also seek to influence and educate policymakers, medical administrators, and trainees about this important subject. As noted previously, patients highly value the interpersonal relationship with their surgeon. Continuity of care is also essential for good patient outcomes [58]. Surgical continuity can be maintained with detailed, structured handoffs, but an interpersonal relationship with built trust cannot be handed off [59].

8.4.4 The Business of Medicine

We have already discussed various models of the doctor-patient relationship, with partnership through shared decision-making typically at the center of establishing trust. Shutzberg proposes a counterpoint that the aggressive influence of business-motivated financial gain in healthcare disempowers both patient and doctor [60]. This is an overly pessimistic view of the American healthcare system, initially proposed as the “age of bureaucratic parsimony,” though it may not always translate to the desired one-on-one interaction in a clinical consultation [61]. Nonetheless, corporate ownership and the cost of healthcare are growing so rapidly that all surgeons will need to recognize how these factors affects their patients and practice [62]. A core principle of practicing medicine and surgery has always been the individual doctor-patient relationship; this should always be shaped by the people in the relationship with the good and well-being of the patient in mind. Physicians have historically been able to design their practice models and schedules to serve this goal, without pressure to meet standardized patient or procedural volume metrics that fail to recognize the inherent individuality of both doctor and patient. Additionally, the corporate application in some cases of the generic label “provider” to physicians reflects a lack of respect for such highly trained professionals and the patients they care for and can, in fact, be demoralizing [63]. In response to the power that government, insurance, pharmaceutical companies, corporations, and healthcare organizations wield, physicians and patients should consider each other comrades in solidarity while navigating or resisting these forces.

One excellent example of such advocacy is against surprise billing practices identified in surgical practices in 2020 [64]. Surprise billing involves an insurance company charging higher “out-of-network” costs to the patient despite the patient undergoing a procedure at an “in-network” facility with an “in-network” surgeon. This practice was also prevalent in emergency visits or transportation, where patients are unable to make financially based choices [65]. Published description of these practices and *advocacy led by surgeons* culminated in the “No Surprises Act,” a federal bill that capped these medical charges, protecting patients. If surgeons recognized these industry dynamics better and advocated for their patients, perhaps it would facilitate developing the solidarity and trust with patients that Shutzberg proposes [66]. And even further, ensuring an equitable and fair surgical patient experience increases the likelihood of a patient placing trust in the surgeon for their next preoperative evaluation.

Because some financial relationships with the potential for conflict of interest are unavoidable, Fadlallah et al. advocate for greater transparency in situations where physicians and private interests are intertwined [67]. This is required in professional educational lecture settings and research proposals, but these disclosures are not readily available to the public. This is similarly stated in the AMA Code of Ethics that physicians “disclose any financial and other factors that could affect the patient’s care,” yet physicians may not be fully aware of how their patients and their practice are influenced [13].

8.4.5 Physician Burnout

Physician burnout is a well-described phenomenon that has come into clearer focus since the turn of the century and was further exacerbated by the COVID-19 pandemic. Today, medical administrative leaders, including the American Medical

Association, US Surgeon General, and Accreditation Council for Graduate Medical Education (postgraduate medical education accreditation body) consider physician burnout a significant issue. We have already discussed administrative burdens associated with care delivery; these are recognized as significant contributors to burnout. A focus on burnout has led to many policy changes, including the well-known 80-hour work week restriction for residents [68].

Surgical disciplines were especially targeted for the highest work hour responsibilities, high-stress environments, and hierarchical structure. Yet some of these rigors are intertwined with surgical values—availability for patient need, care continuity, risk, and exceptional levels of responsibility. These are common elements from which surgeons derive fulfillment and joy, leading them to choose this challenging profession in the first place [69–71]. This complicates interventions to improve quality of life and decrease burnout. That is, surgical practice and training are inherently physically and emotionally demanding endeavors; to think otherwise is a misconception. Aligning expectations with the realities of the profession, while simultaneously embracing opportunities to reduce burnout without sacrificing core values, seems like a balanced approach. The longest, most demanding days can also be the most rewarding and, anecdotally, the best opportunities to build trust with patients. Patients often comment when they perceive their surgeons to be working hard, even if not directly on their case, whether during late nights in the hospital, long clinic discussions, or in anticipation of a long case in the operating room. Patients desire a well-rested and clear-headed surgeon, but also one who will go the extra mile for them in their time of need, regardless of surgeon comfort or inconvenience.

8.5 Trust and Humanism

Walking through a postoperative recovery room, the humanistic concept of human flourishing feels quite distant. Anesthesia is disorienting for hours following a procedure, and surgery almost always results in some pain and sometimes results in outright suffering. Patients slowly regain their humanity and vitality as they recover, and many face new postoperative realities ahead of them. Each of those patients knowingly accepted these challenges because they trusted the caregivers and the care process.

In our opening case example of a patient with a narrowed airway, a decision to undergo surgery carries both great risk and the potential for great reward. A dilation of the airway can transform a patient from someone who can barely move from their bed, to one who can comfortably walk miles with their partner or children, or readily accomplish required tasks in their workplace. While this can be a routine procedure for subspecialists, the patient and surgeon must, nonetheless, weigh benefits against real potential surgical risks and complications. Established trust is the key to navigating this journey. Together, patient and surgeon can determine what best constitutes individualized flourishing. The role of guiding patients through these challenging decisions, while also enacting and accomplishing the surgical treatment plan, is at the core of surgical professionalism and medical humanism. Indeed, among the most consequential and fulfilling surgeon-patient exchanges is a preoperative visit that closes with: "We will take good care of you." and,"I know you will. I trust you."

References

1. Berges AJ, Lina IA, Chen L, Ospino R, Davis R, Hillel AT. Delayed diagnosis of idiopathic subglottic stenosis. Laryngoscope. 2022;132(2):413–8. https://doi.org/10.1002/lary.29783. Epub 2021 Aug 9. PMID: 34369599; PMCID: PMC8742746.
2. Damico Smith C, Nanda N, Bonnet K, Schlundt D, Anderson C, Fernandes-Taylor S, Gelbard A, Francis DO. Navigating pathways to diagnosis in idiopathic subglottic stenosis: a qualitative study. Laryngoscope. 2024;134(2):815–24. https://doi.org/10.1002/lary.31023. Epub 2023 Sept 23. PMID: 37740907.
3. Montori VM, Ruissen MM, Hargraves IG, Brito JP, Kunneman M. Shared decision-making as a method of care. BMJ Evid Based Med. 2023;28(4):213–7. https://doi.org/10.1136/bmjebm-2022-112068. Epub 2022 Dec 2. PMID: 36460328; PMCID: PMC10423463.
4. Hargraves IG, Montori VM, Brito JP, Kunneman M, Shaw K, LaVecchia C, Wilson M, Walker L, Thorsteinsdottir B. Purposeful SDM: a problem-based approach to caring for patients with shared decision making. Patient Educ Couns. 2019;102(10):1786–92. https://doi.org/10.1016/j.pec.2019.07.020. Epub 2019 July 19. PMID: 31353170; PMCID: PMC6717012.
5. Schattner A. The essence of humanistic medicine. QJM. 2020;113(1):3–4. https://doi.org/10.1093/qjmed/hcz155. PMID: 31228249.
6. Lee Roze des Ordons A, de Groot JM, Rosenal T, Viceer N, Nixon L. How clinicians integrate humanism in their clinical workplace—'Just trying to put myself in their human being shoes'. Perspect Med Educ. 2018;7(5):318–24. https://doi.org/10.1007/s40037-018-0455-4. PMID: 30298438; PMCID: PMC6191400.
7. Spadaro G, Gangl K, Van Prooijen JW, Van Lange PAM, Mosso CO. Enhancing feelings of security: how institutional trust promotes interpersonal trust. PLoS One. 2020;15(9):e0237934. https://doi.org/10.1371/journal.pone.0237934. PMID: 32916694; PMCID: PMC7486136.
8. Govier T. Self-trust, autonomy, and self-esteem. Hypatia. 1993;8(1):99–120. http://www.jstor.org/stable/3810303
9. Hall MA, Dugan E, Zheng B, Mishra AK. Trust in physicians and medical institutions: what is it, can it be measured, and does it matter? Milbank Q. 2001;79(4):613–39. https://doi.org/10.1111/1468-0009.00223. PMID: 11789119; PMCID: PMC2751209.
10. McGeer V. Trust, hope and empowerment. Austral J Philos. 86(2):237–54. https://doi.org/10.1080/00048400801886413.
11. McLeod C. Trust. The Stanford Encyclopedia of Philosophy (Fall 2023 edition). https://plato.stanford.edu/archives/fall2023/entries/trust/
12. Scheman N. Trust and trustworthiness. In: The Routledge handbook of trust and philosophy. London: Routledge; 2020. ISBN 9781315542294.
13. Patient-physician relationships. AMA code of medical ethics. 2016. https://code-medical-ethics.ama-assn.org/
14. Statement on principles. American College of Surgeons 2016 Apr 12. https://www.facs.org/about-acs/statements/statements-on-principles/
15. Davey B, Sinha R, Lee JH, Gauthier M, Flores G. Social determinants of health and outcomes for children and adults with congenital heart disease: a systematic review. Pediatr Res. 2021;89(2):275–94. https://doi.org/10.1038/s41390-020-01196-6. Epub 2020 Oct 17. PMID: 33069160.

16. Wilder ME, Kulie P, Jensen C, Levett P, Blanchard J, Dominguez LW, Portela M, Srivastava A, Li Y, McCarthy ML. The impact of social determinants of health on medication adherence: a systematic review and meta-analysis. J Gen Intern Med. 2021;36(5):1359–70. https://doi.org/10.1007/s11606-020-06447-0. Epub 2021 Jan 29. PMID: 33515188; PMCID: PMC8131473.
17. Carter AJ. Therapeutic trust. Philos Psychol. 2024;37(1):38–61. https://doi.org/10.1080/09515089.2022.2058925.
18. Schwarze ML, Bradley CT, Brasel KJ. Surgical "buy-in": the contractual relationship between surgeons and patients that influences decisions regarding life-supporting therapy. Crit Care Med. 2010;38(3):843–8. https://doi.org/10.1097/CCM.0b013e3181cc466b. PMID: 20048678; PMCID: PMC3042894.
19. Skowron KB, Angelos P. Surgical informed consent revisited: time to revise the routine? World J Surg. 2017;41(1):1–4. https://doi.org/10.1007/s00268-016-3715-7. PMID: 27637605.
20. Nabozny MJ, Kruser JM, Steffens NM, Pecanac KE, Brasel KJ, Chittenden EH, Cooper Z, McKneally MF, Schwarze ML. Patient-reported limitations to surgical buy-in: a qualitative study of patients facing high-risk surgery. Ann Surg. 2017;265(1):97–102. https://doi.org/10.1097/SLA.0000000000001645. PMID: 28009732; PMCID: PMC4949135.
21. Nguyen AL, Schwei RJ, Zhao YQ, Rathouz PJ, Jacobs EA. What matters when it comes to trust in one's physician: race/ethnicity, sociodemographic factors, and/or access to and experiences with health care? Health Equity. 2020;4(1):280–9. https://doi.org/10.1089/heq.2019.0101. PMID: 34095698; PMCID: PMC8175262.
22. Hogikyan ND, Kana LA, Shuman AG, Firn JI. Patient perceptions of trust formation in the surgeon-patient relationship: a thematic analysis. Patient Educ Couns. 2021;104(9):2338–43. https://doi.org/10.1016/j.pec.2021.02.002. Epub 2021 Feb 5. PMID: 33583655.
23. Lu LY, Sheikholeslami N, Alokozai A, Eppler SL, Kamal RN. The role of patient research in patient trust in their physician. J Hand Surg Am. 2019;44(7):617.e1–9. https://doi.org/10.1016/j.jhsa.2018.09.007. Epub 2018 Oct 23. PMID: 30366736.
24. Blakely K, Karanicolas PJ, Wright FC, Gotlib CL. Optimistic honesty: understanding surgeon and patient perspectives on hopeful communication in pancreatic cancer care. HPB (Oxford). 2017;19(7):611–9. https://doi.org/10.1016/j.hpb.2017.04.001. Epub 2017 May 17. PMID: 28528268.
25. Hillen MA, Onderwater AT, van Zwieten MC, de Haes HC, Smets EM. Disentangling cancer patients' trust in their oncologist: a qualitative study. Psychooncology. 2012;21(4):392–9. https://doi.org/10.1002/pon.1910. Epub 2011 Jan 30. PMID: 21280138.
26. Hamelin ND, Nikolis A, Armano J, Harris PG, Brutus JP. Evaluation of factors influencing confidence and trust in the patient-physician relationship: a survey of patient in a hand clinic. Chir Main. 2012;31(2):83–90. https://doi.org/10.1016/j.main.2012.01.005. Epub 2012 Feb 3. PMID: 22365321.
27. Whitney RL, White AEC, Rosenberg AS, Kravitz RL, Kim KK. Trust and shared decision-making among individuals with multiple myeloma: a qualitative study. Cancer Med. 2021;10(22):8040–57. https://doi.org/10.1002/cam4.4322. Epub 2021 Oct 5. PMID: 34608770; PMCID: PMC8607252.
28. Lincoln TE, Buddadhumaruk P, Arnold RM, Scheunemann LP, Ernecoff NC, Chang CH, Carson SS, Hough CL, Curtis JR, Anderson W, Steingrub J, Peterson MW, Lo B, Matthay MA, White DB. Association between shared decision-making during family meetings and surrogates' trust in their ICU physician. Chest. 2023;163(5):1214–24. https://doi.org/10.1016/j.chest.2022.10.028. Epub 2022 Nov 3. PMID: 36336000; PMCID: PMC10258434.
29. Grad R, Légaré F, Bell NR, Dickinson JA, Singh H, Moore AE, Kasperavicius D, Kretschmer KL. Shared decision making in preventive health care: what it is; what it is not. Can Fam Physician. 2017;63(9):682–4. PMID: 28904031; PMCID: PMC5597010.
30. Faiman B, Tariman JD. Shared decision making: improving patient outcomes by understanding the benefits of and barriers to effective communication. Clin J Oncol Nurs. 2019;23(5):540–2. https://doi.org/10.1188/19.CJON.540-542. PMID: 31538972.

31. Forner D, Noel CW, Shuman AG, Hong P, Corsten M, Rac VE, Pieterse AH, Goldstein D. Shared decision-making in head and neck surgery: a review. JAMA Otolaryngol Head Neck Surg. 2020;146(9):839–44. https://doi.org/10.1001/jamaoto.2020.1601. PMID: 32701131.
32. Dang BN, Westbrook RA, Njue SM, Giordano TP. Building trust and rapport early in the new doctor-patient relationship: a longitudinal qualitative study. BMC Med Educ. 2017;17(1):32. https://doi.org/10.1186/s12909-017-0868-5. PMID: 28148254; PMCID: PMC5288896.
33. Fritz Z, Holton R. Too much medicine: not enough trust? J Med Ethics. 2019;45(1):31–5. https://doi.org/10.1136/medethics-2018-104866. Epub 2018 Oct 26. PMID: 30367013; PMCID: PMC6327867.
34. Occelli P, Mougeot F, Robelet M, Buchet-Poyau K, Touzet S, Michel P. Feelings of trust and of safety are related facets of the patient's experience in surgery: a descriptive qualitative study in 80 patients. J Patient Saf. 2022;18(5):415–20. https://doi.org/10.1097/PTS.0000000000000950. Epub 2021 Dec 17. PMID: 35948291.
35. Sah S, Fagerlin A, Ubel P. Effect of physician disclosure of specialty bias on patient trust and treatment choice. Proc Natl Acad Sci USA. 2016;113(27):7465–9. https://doi.org/10.1073/pnas.1604908113. Epub 2016 June 20. PMID: 27325783; PMCID: PMC4941435.
36. Leclercq WK, Keulers BJ, Scheltinga MR, Spauwen PH, van der Wilt GJ. A review of surgical informed consent: past, present, and future. A quest to help patients make better decisions. World J Surg. 2010;34(7):1406–15. https://doi.org/10.1007/s00268-010-0542-0. PMID: 20372902; PMCID: PMC2895877.
37. Palmer BW, Harmell AL. Assessment of healthcare decision-making capacity. Arch Clin Neuropsychol. 2016;31(6):530–40. https://doi.org/10.1093/arclin/acw051. Epub 2016 Aug 22. PMID: 27551024; PMCID: PMC5007079.
38. Barstow C, Shahan B, Roberts M. Evaluating medical decision-making capacity in practice. Am Fam Physician. 2018;98(1):40–6. PMID: 30215955.
39. Ricketts D, Roper T, Rogers B, Phadnis J, Elsayed S, Sokol D. Informed consent: the view from the trenches. Ann R Coll Surg Engl. 2019;101(1):44–9. https://doi.org/10.1308/rcsann.2018.0140. Epub 2018 Oct 5. PMID: 30286630; PMCID: PMC6303806.
40. Courtney MJ. Information about surgery: what does the public want to know? ANZ J Surg. 2001;71(1):24–6. https://doi.org/10.1046/j.1440-1622.2001.02026.x. PMID: 11167593.
41. Gabay G, Bokek-Cohen Y. What do patients want? Surgical informed-consent and patient-centered care – an augmented model of information disclosure. Bioethics. 2020;34(5):467–77. https://doi.org/10.1111/bioe.12703. Epub 2019 Dec 2. PMID: 31788815.
42. Sullivan LS. Trust, risk, and race in American medicine. Hast Cent Rep. 2020;50(1):18–26. https://doi.org/10.1002/hast.1080. PMID: 32068281.
43. Miller F, Miller P. Transgenerational trauma and trust restoration. AMA J Ethics. 2021;23(6):E480–6. https://doi.org/10.1001/amajethics.2021.480. PMID: 34212849.
44. Langerman A, Brelsford KM, Diehl CJ, Harris CR, Stewart TG. Trust as a predictor of patient perceptions regarding overlapping surgery and trainee Independence. Laryngoscope. 2020;130(11):2728–35. https://doi.org/10.1002/lary.28557. Epub 2020 Feb 17. PMID: 32065409.
45. Regenbogen SE, Veenstra CM, Hawley ST, Hendren S, Ward KC, Kato I, Morris AM. The effect of complications on the patient-surgeon relationship after colorectal cancer surgery. Surgery. 2014;155(5):841–50. https://doi.org/10.1016/j.surg.2013.12.011. Epub 2013 Dec 15. PMID: 24787111; PMCID: PMC4254758.
46. Sucher S, Gupta S. The trust crisis. Harv Bus Rev. 2019; https://hbr.org/2019/07/the-trust-crisis.
47. Keslar L. The trust crisis. Proto MGH 2022 Mar 28. https://protomag.com/clinical-care/the-trust-crisis/.
48. Axelrod DA, Goold SD. Maintaining trust in the surgeon-patient relationship: challenges for the new millennium. Arch Surg. 2000;135(1):55–61. https://doi.org/10.1001/archsurg.135.1.55. PMID: 10636348.

49. Kennedy B, Tyson A, Funk C. Americans' trust in scientists, other groups declines. Pew Research Center. 2022 Feb 15. https://www.pewresearch.org/science/2022/02/15/americans-trust-in-scientists-other-groups-declines/
50. Budd J. Burnout related to electronic health record use in primary care. J Prim Care Community Health, 101177/21501319231166921. 2023;14:21501319231166921. PMID: 37073905; PMCID: PMC10134123.
51. Muhiyaddin R, Elfadl A, Mohamed E, Shah Z, Alam T, Abd-Alrazaq A, Househ M. Electronic health records and physician burnout: a scoping review. Stud Health Technol Inform. 2022;289:481–4. https://doi.org/10.3233/SHTI210962. PMID: 35062195.
52. New HHS Study shows 63-fold increase in medicare telehealth utilization during the pandemic. CMS.gov Newsroom. 2021 Dec 3. https://www.cms.gov/newsroom/press-releases/new-hhs-study-shows-63-fold-increase-medicare-telehealth-utilization-during-pandemic
53. Hogikyan ND, Shuman AG. Otolaryngologists and the doctor-patient relationship during a pandemic. Otolaryngol Head Neck Surg. 2020;163(1):63–4. https://doi.org/10.1177/0194599820922990. Epub 2020 Apr 28. PMID: 32340553.
54. Buchanan S, Peixoto C, Belanger C, Archibald D, Bjerre L, Fitzsimon J. Investigating patient experience, satisfaction, and trust in an integrated virtual care (IVC) model: a cross-sectional survey. Ann Fam Med. 2023;21(4):338–40. https://doi.org/10.1370/afm.2978. Epub 2023 Mar 21. PMID: 36944507; PMCID: PMC10365871.
55. Tam S, Neslund-Dudas C, Barrett AM, Barrow LCJ, Fridman I, Kinlaw AC, Puviindran P, Royce TJ, Smith AB, Stein JN, Wood WA, Elston Lafata J. The perceived usability of virtual visits among black adults' receiving oncology care: a qualitative analysis. Oncologist. 2024;29(2):e237–47. https://doi.org/10.1093/oncolo/oyad260. PMID: 37756655; PMCID: PMC10836309.
56. O'Connor AL, Shmelev A, Shettig A, Santucci NM, Bray J, Bazarian A, Orenstein SB, Nikolian VC. Assessing patient-reported experiences for in-person and telemedicine-based preoperative evaluations. Telemed J E Health. 2024;30(2):472–9. https://doi.org/10.1089/tmj.2023.0089. Epub 2023 Aug 25. PMID: 37624627.
57. Katta MH, Shao CC, Jones B, Nehemiah A, Krouse R, Ko C, Chu DI. The role of telemedicine in building trust: an evolution of the patient-surgeon relationship. Am J Surg. 2023;S0002-9610(23):00614–1. https://doi.org/10.1016/j.amjsurg.2023.11.010. Epub ahead of print. PMID: 38007368.
58. Justiniano CF, Xu Z, Becerra AZ, Aquina CT, Boodry CI, Temple LK, Fleming FJ. Effect of care continuity on mortality of patients readmitted after colorectal surgery. Br J Surg. 2019;106(5):636–44. https://doi.org/10.1002/bjs.11078. Epub 2019 Feb 1. PMID: 30706462.
59. Koea JB, Srinivasa S, Hundal H. Provision of acute general surgery: a systematic review of models of care. J Trauma Acute Care Surg. 2014;76(1):219–25. https://doi.org/10.1097/TA.0b013e3182a92481. PMID: 24368384.
60. Shutzberg M. The doctor as parent, partner, provider… or comrade? Distribution of power in past and present models of the doctor-patient relationship. Health Care Anal. 2021;29(3):231–48. https://doi.org/10.1007/s10728-021-00432-2. Epub 2021 Apr 27. PMID: 33905025; PMCID: PMC8322008.
61. Siegler M. The progression of medicine. From physician paternalism to patient autonomy to bureaucratic parsimony. Arch Intern Med. 1985;145(4):713–5. https://doi.org/10.1001/archinte.145.4.713. PMID: 3885894.
62. Christou CD, Athanasiadou EC, Tooulias AI, Tzamalis A, Tsoulfas G. The process of estimating the cost of surgery: providing a practical framework for surgeons. Int J Health Plann Manag. 2022;37(4):1926–40. https://doi.org/10.1002/hpm.3431. Epub 2022 Feb 21. PMID: 35191067.
63. Goroll AH. Eliminating the term primary care "provider": consequences of language for the future of primary care. JAMA. 2016;315(17):1833–4. https://doi.org/10.1001/jama.2016.2329. PMID: 27031172.

64. Chhabra KR, Sheetz KH, Nuliyalu U, Dekhne MS, Ryan AM, Dimick JB. Out-of-network bills for privately insured patients undergoing elective surgery with in-network primary surgeons and facilities. JAMA. 2020;323(6):538–47. https://doi.org/10.1001/jama.2019.21463. PMID: 32044941; PMCID: PMC7042888.
65. Colla C. Surprise billing-a flashpoint for major policy issues in health care. JAMA. 2021;325(8):715–6. https://doi.org/10.1001/jama.2020.26779. PMID: 33620413.
66. Thom DH, Hall MA, Pawlson LG. Measuring patients' trust in physicians when assessing quality of care. Health Aff (Millwood). 2004;23(4):124–32. https://doi.org/10.1377/hlthaff.23.4.124. PMID: 15318572.
67. Fadlallah R, Nas H, Naamani D, El-Jardali F, Hammoura I, Al-Khaled L, Brax H, Kahale L, Akl EA. Knowledge, beliefs and attitudes of patients and the general public towards the interactions of physicians with the pharmaceutical and the device industry: a systematic review. PLoS One. 2016;11(8):e0160540. https://doi.org/10.1371/journal.pone.0160540. PMID: 27556929; PMCID: PMC4996522.
68. Chi D, Chen AD, Wu WW, Chattha A, Lee BT, Lin SJ. Evaluating the impact of ACGME resident duty hour restrictions on patient outcomes for bilateral breast reductions. Plast Reconstr Surg Glob Open. 2023;11(2):e4820. https://doi.org/10.1097/GOX.0000000000004820. PMID: 36761011; PMCID: PMC9904753.
69. Coleman JR, Tracy TB, Kalamar CL, McNicoll CF, Ryan R. Shift work surgery: loss of continuity or sensible balance of responsibility? Am Coll Surg Bull. 2019 Aug 1. https://www.facs.org/for-medical-professionals/news-publications/news-and-articles/bulletin/2019/08/shift-work-surgery-loss-of-continuity-or-sensible-balance-of-responsibility/
70. Coverdill JE, Alseidi A, Borgstrom DC, Dent DL, Dumire RD, Fryer J, Hartranft TH, Holsten SB, Nelson MT, Shabahang M, Sherman S, Termuhlen PM, Woods RJ, Mellinger JD. Professionalism in the twilight zone: a multicenter, mixed-methods study of shift transition dynamics in surgical residencies. Acad Med. 2016;91(11 Association of American Medical Colleges Learn Serve Lead, Proceedings of the 55th Annual Research in Medical Education Sessions):S31–6. https://doi.org/10.1097/ACM.0000000000001358. PMID: 27779507.
71. Hughes D, Hanson MN, Alseidi A, Romanelli J, Vassiliou M, Feldman LS, Asbun H. Factors influencing surgeon well-being: qualitatively exploring the joy of surgery. Surg Endosc. 2023;37(8):6464–75. https://doi.org/10.1007/s00464-023-10135-5. Epub 2023 May 23. PMID: 37221414; PMCID: PMC10204656.

Chapter 9
Operating on the Critically Ill: The Need for Shared Decision-Making in a Technologically Sophisticated Healthcare Environment

Katherine Bakke

9.1 Introduction

Critically ill patients, usually being cared for by intensivists in an intensive care unit (ICU) or being seen by emergency physicians in the emergency department (ED), can have or develop a life-threatening diagnosis for which the primary treatment is surgery. However, the risks of surgery can be very high, whereas the benefits of a successful surgery, given the patient's underlying illnesses or functional status, might be quite marginal or debatable.

The success of a surgery is dependent on the goal of the operation—be it to alleviate pain, help a patient live longer, or prevent disability. Surgery is not a panacea, and it is increasingly clear that surgery carries long-term ramifications on a patient's longevity and functional status. Take, for example, patients with malignant small bowel obstruction due to disseminated cancer. These patients are living with a terminal disease, but advances in chemotherapy, radiation, and immunotherapy have helped many live longer than ever before. However, patients undergoing surgery for a malignant small bowel obstruction face a mortality rate of nearly three times that of patients with small bowel obstruction due to benign disease [1]. Furthermore, only 45% of patients with malignant small bowel obstruction who underwent surgery were able to achieve the stated goal of the operation, which was the ability to tolerate solid food postoperatively [2]. Elderly patients living independently prior to an emergency operation face a 12% risk of in-hospital death, 14% risk of death within a year, and 10% risk of discharging permanently to a facility [3]. For patients who are already considered frail, this risk is higher [4]. By these metrics, surgery can help many, but not all, patients. Thus, whether surgery is in the patient's best

K. Bakke (✉)
Division of Acute Care and Regional General Surgery, Department of Surgery, University of Wisconsin School of Medicine and Public Health, Madison, WI, USA
e-mail: bakke@surgery.wisc.edu

F. Jotterand, C. Bosco (eds.), *Fostering Humanism in Surgery*, New Paradigms in Healthcare, https://doi.org/10.1007/978-3-031-82771-6_9

interest can be uncertain. The surgeon's decision to recommend surgery or not can be extremely difficult, and the criteria that a surgeon uses to make that recommendation are often unclear.

This chapter explores the issues and the evidence involved in the decision-making process for a critically ill patient with an acute surgical condition. Personal vignettes are used to illustrate some of the issues involved. I first review the literature that attempts to examine the morbidity and mortality outcomes of this unique patient population—medically complex, critically ill patients facing a surgical emergency. I consider the surgeons' perspective to these clinical situations, which is informed and influenced by the unique beliefs and values that define the culture of surgery. I attempt to describe how patients and/or their surrogates see themselves when making such life-or-death decisions. The chapter concludes by discussing shared decision-making and how shared decision-making remedies many of the communication problems surgeons face in making these difficult clinical judgments.

9.2 The Situation

In an increasingly technologically sophisticated medical landscape, machines, medications, and invasive monitoring systems can support the most critically ill patient through an acute medical illness. Surgeons, however, are frequently consulted when life-threatening complications arise and the clinical situation deteriorates. Examples include when abdominal compartment syndrome sends a patient with acute pancreatitis into multisystem organ failure, or a patient with metastatic colon cancer on second-line chemotherapy becomes septic due to bowel perforation, or a patient with cirrhosis and portal hypertension suffers a mesenteric thrombus and develops intestinal ischemia.

The mortality of these conditions, and others like them, is high in these fragile patients regardless of intervention. The surgeon must weigh the potential benefits of surgery against the possibility that surgical intervention will add to the patient's suffering, as well as their loved ones, regardless of whether the patient lives or dies.

I admit, when I receive pages asking for a STAT surgical consult for an acute abdomen in a patient who is critically ill, I feel a sense of dread. The variables for prognostication are many and difficult to parse. The probability that death is near for the person I am about to meet is often quite high, regardless of my actions. The situation at the bedside can feel like I am being asked to decide if the patient will get a "chance" to live.

When I walk into a patient's room and introduce myself as the surgeon, I see the pleading faces of family members with the wordless imploration to "do something," and the patient appearing helpless and clearly seeking relief from their suffering. My hands itch to do something to help, for that is what I have been trained to do. The operating room is safe—the safest place in the hospital, I often tell patients—and it is only natural for me to want to run to the safest place when facing such a threat.

In a culture where "life" holds many definitions—the presence of a heartbeat, maintenance of metabolic homeostasis, the opportunity to achieve one's fullest potential, and the ability to love and be loved—I struggle to know if my efforts in operating on the most critically ill are honoring life or doing harm. As a surgeon, I literally "do things" to patients, and as such, I am the gatekeeper to a technology that has the potential to be lifesaving. If I withhold that knowledge, skill, and technology, am I forsaking my responsibility to others? Or, by operating in dire circumstances, am I simply performing, what we cynically called in residency, "the death operation"? Research has attempted to rationalize these decisions with statistics and risk calculators, useful but incomplete tools when deciding to operate in a critical situation. These tools ignore the ethical stresses that surgeons like myself, as well as patients and their families, face in the crucial moment of deciding to go, or not to go, to the operating room. In employing shared decision-making techniques and strategies, I have learned to ask, just because a surgeon "can" operate, does it mean that a surgeon "should" operate?

9.3 The Data

Patients who require emergency operations have higher rates of complications and mortality compared to those patients who undergo operations electively. This is an objectively known, and clinically intuitive, fact. Less is known about the morbidity and mortality facing patients who are already extremely sick and acutely in need of an operation. As medicine advances and allows physicians to care for critically ill patients with medications and machines with success, this knowledge gap is of increasing importance. Briggs et al. at the University of Pittsburgh, the birthplace of critical care medicine, have studied this ultra-vulnerable patient population. Over the course of 6 years, 911 medical intensive care (MICU) patients required surgical consultations, which is, admittedly, only a small portion (8%) of all MICU admissions. Of this cohort, 411 patients (45%) required an operative intervention. 186 of these patients (20% of the total number of patients receiving surgical consultation) required emergent abdominal surgery. Common pathologies included Clostridium difficile colitis, bowel obstruction, ischemic bowel, peptic ulcer disease, pancreatitis, and cholecystitis. Overall mortality for these patients requiring abdominal operations was 37%, whereas the mortality rate was 16% for all patients admitted to the MICU during the same period. They also noted that 26 patients had pathology amenable to surgery but did not undergo an operation; 100% of these patients died. Briggs et al. remark "It is important for surgeons to recognize the patients who are unlikely to be rescued to avoid nonbeneficial procedures while also maintaining a low threshold for early intervention in the population that has potential for rescue" [5].

But, how do we do that?

There is objective data that can aid in these decisions. In the same study, Briggs et al. found that certain procedures were associated with higher mortality than others. For example, a bowel resection had a mortality rate of 42%, whereas an appendectomy and cholecystectomy were much lower (0% and 11% respectively). Additionally, factors like delay in diagnosis, preoperative need for hemodialysis, and elevated bilirubin levels increased a patient's odds of mortality. Of note, age contributed only slightly to increased odds of death; physiologic disturbances such as organ failure and systems issues like delay in diagnosis contributed more to a patient's death than his or her age.

Due to the increasing complexity of medical illness, preexisting comorbidities, and the physiologic disturbances of surgical disease, risk calculators have been developed to aid surgeons in decision-making on whether to offer an operation to a critically ill patient. Huckaby et al. examined 150 patients and the 17 surgeons involved in their care to see if risk calculators and surgeon estimates regarding mortality and various complications (e.g., renal failure and need for hemodialysis) were comparable. This study found that both surgeons and risk calculators underestimated overall mortality [6]. Other studies have demonstrated that both "objective" scoring systems and physician prognostication are "overly optimistic" [7].

Survival is not the only factor surgeons and patients need to consider. What does life look like after survival from critical illness? One study demonstrated that 32% of Medicare beneficiaries undergoing an emergency operation on the first or second day of a hospital admission were, at 1 year, either dead or had experienced permanent loss of independence [3]. Post-intensive care syndrome (PICS) describes the multifaceted mental and physical disturbances that linger after an ICU illness and is an emerging topic of study. PICS includes muscle weakness limiting one's ability to independently function in activities of daily living, cognitive impairments affecting memory and executive functioning, and mental health disease including anxiety, depression, and post-traumatic stress disorder. Additional components of PICS include difficulty swallowing, metabolic dysfunction, sleep disorders, residual fatigue, persistent pain, and bone loss leading to skeletal fragility. How long PICS lasts is difficult to define and does not always correlate with age. Generally, a patient's frailty prior to critical illness portends a "reduced chance of recovery compared to a previously healthy patient" [8]. A patient's social support is crucial to recovery and re-establishing a life outside the ICU, and is often an underrecognized component to a patient's success for recovery after hospitalization [9].

The survival of critically ill patients undergoing emergency surgery is better than the estimates of many experienced surgeons. I anticipated a higher mortality rate for MICU patients undergoing emergency surgical interventions. I think of the patients that I did not operate on—who, as the study says, had a 100% mortality rate—and wonder if I should have taken the chance to save their life and proceeded to the operating room. I also think about the patients on whom I have operated, patients who survived the surgery itself but faced years-long recovery and permanent loss of function. I recall one patient who survived his emergency operation for mesenteric ischemia but then developed nonhealing wounds on both legs and required bilateral above-knee amputations, rendering him wheelchair-bound. His wife told me she wanted him to be able to dress up as Santa Claus at their annual holiday party. The patient's nurse repeatedly asked me to address "goals of care," as the patient had voiced to her his wish to die. When I spoke to the patient himself, he was withdrawn and hardly engaged with me.

When we know our operations can create this type of suffering, what are we to do? The guiding ethical principle for all physicians—first, do no harm—becomes much more nuanced.

9.4 The Surgeon

Although the demographic makeup of practicing surgeons is diversifying, surgical culture—those values that mold an individual surgeon and unite surgeons in an exclusive fraternity—has remained relatively static. Francis Moore, a surgeon-scientist who studied metabolism in the surgical patient, wrote, "the practice of surgery is the assumption of complete responsibility for the welfare of the patient suffering from these [surgical] diseases" [10]. From this concept of "complete responsibility" emerge attitudes, beliefs, and perceptions that surgeons bring to the decision of whether to operate on a critically ill patient.

To describe the "inner deliberations" of surgeons treating critically ill patients, Kulkarni et al. interviewed 40 surgeons, asking them to "think aloud" about memorable cases during which they did, or did not, operate on a critically ill patient. In a pictorial representation of themes that contributed to a surgeon's decision-making, "surgeon factors" such as individual characteristics and intrinsic motivation were notably equal to, or larger than, patient factors or the patient's surgical problem. In other words, the surgeon's own beliefs and values factor largely, and sometimes dominate, the formulation of a patient's treatment.

Kulkarni et al. found that all surgeons first collected data on the patient—vital signs, comorbidities, lab values, exam findings, and imaging studies—to formulate a diagnosis. "All surgeons integrated their assessments by determining the likelihood of immediate reversibility, survival, and the patient's return to pre-existing functional status." Surgeons then filtered this information through their own lens: "they valued their cumulative experience in providing 'wisdom' about when not to operate and cited formative experiences early in their career that continue to influence their decision making." Additionally, "surgeons sought diagnostic certainty (identifying the diagnosis when otherwise unclear), therapeutic simplicity (straightforward management, a problem that is 'very easily fixed'), and a smooth resolution of cases (when patients 'do okay without any major complications')." To a lesser extent, surgeons spoke about societal norms—or "collective expectations of how one ought to behave"—that influenced their decisions. Surgeons felt pressure to "do everything" due to "unrealistic expectations of what we can do;" implicitly, those expecting the surgeon to do everything are the patient and their family [11].

Anthropologist Joan Cassell elaborates on the idea that surgeons possess some sort of divine healing power, in *Expected Miracles*:

> Performing surgery involves a dreadful power, that of life and death. Working a miracle is its positive aspect: doing something that rescues a person from death. "Playing God" is the negative aspect: the accusation hurled by angry and frightened patients and families when surgeons refuse or are unable to perform a procedure that will save someone from death, or when they refuse to stop saving that person from an impending and inevitable death. I heard few surgeons speak of this aspect of their profession.... I suspect surgeons rarely discuss the metaphysical aspects of surgery with each other. It's frightening to think of oneself as possessing such awesome power; it puts a heavy weight on someone who, however arrogant and egotistical, knows his abilities are fully, and merely, human. [12]

As a surgeon, I found myself nodding my head and murmuring "uh-huh's" while reading Kulkarni's research and Cassell's anthropologic observations. When on call, I rejoice when there is a straightforward clinical problem to fix, even if fixing it proves to be a technical challenge. It is easy to take an elderly patient to the OR with a perforated gastric ulcer who was otherwise healthy a few days before their presentation to the emergency department. It is much harder to take a malnourished, intubated patient on stress-dose steroids and pressors to the operating room with the same issue. While I know I can technically do the surgery, I imagine the suffering the patient will experience in their long course to recovery, not to mention the loss of independence if they leave the hospital. I think about all the literature that says the elderly value maintaining independence over longevity. Once again, I ask myself, does my technical ability to perform the surgery mean that I should perform the surgery? My surgical skills, modern medicine, and the human body itself have limits. Sometimes my drive to heal falls short, and patients end up in a limbo of marginal health with revolving medical admissions, chronic pain, GI distress, and complex wound care from the "good" I attempted to do. I suspect some people would define this as a fate worse than the death they would have suffered had surgery not been done.

9.5 The Patient

We frequently extrapolate findings from the literature on the values that individuals with chronic illness place on quality-of-life issues to the critically ill patient population. Patients living with chronic medical conditions, such as COPD, cancer, or congestive heart failure, state they are less likely to choose a treatment with a high likelihood of an adverse outcome. Additionally, fewer patients would choose a treatment when the likelihood of an adverse outcome involved functional or cognitive impairment than when the adverse outcome was death [13]. In other words, many patients think that it takes more than the fact of being alive to make life worth living.

However, little is known about the patient's experience after emergency surgery. Two studies have been performed assessing the patient's experience after an emergency operation. Sokas et al. interviewed 31 patients who had survived for 3 months after an emergency operation. Themes that emerged from these interviews focused on the confusion, fear, and lack of recollection of the moments prior to surgery.

Patients described being "stunned by the rapid onset of illness" and that they had "no choice" but to have surgery. Their goal was to "prolong life" and "notably absent from their 'in-the-moment' thinking was the potential aftermath of surgery including physical and cognitive decline, loss of independence, or nursing home care." Most patients interviewed (81%) in this study, it is important to note, were discharged to their home [14].

Ho et al. interviewed 11 patients and 4 caregivers 1 year after a patient had undergone an emergency operation. Common themes from this study included the importance of family support to a patient's recovery, a desire to "get back to normal," and accepting that some symptoms, such as pain, impaired mobility, or irregular GI function, would persist. However, patients did not see surgery as a "choice" but rather the "only rational option to treat a severe symptom or life-threatening illness." Patients had few recollections of a discussion with a surgeon about the decision to have surgery. Interestingly, they often had vivid memories of conflicting recommendations from clinicians on the best course of treatment [9].

9.6 The Family

Frequently, critically ill patients are unable to make decisions about their care secondary to mental status changes related to their underlying disease process or their associated treatment. Thus, surrogates, be it family or friends, appointed by the patient to make decisions on their behalf (or simply because they are the "next of kin") are asked to make decisions regarding operative management when the patient falls ill with a surgical disease.

The use of surrogates is intended to preserve patient autonomy. Lilley et al. performed a qualitative study in which 19 surrogates were interviewed about how they viewed their role as a surrogate decision-maker. Two archetypal roles that surrogates assumed emerged. One role was that of a "preference advocate, who focused on the patient's values" and relied on the medical team to make recommendations that aligned with the patient's values; however, it was not always clear how the surrogate communicated the patient's values to these decision-makers or verified that treatment recommendations had considered these values. The other role was that of a "clinical facilitator," who focused on the patient's clinical status and believed their ultimate responsibility was to ensure the patient receives the highest quality care. All surrogates who were interviewed remarked that they never received instructions or guidance from clinicians on what their role as a surrogate entailed or how to approach decisions; "as a result, they constructed their understanding of the surrogate role primarily from personal experiences and perceptions." Both archetypes have their ethical pitfalls:

> Clinical facilitators justified decisions to overrule the patient's preferences if they believed that a different course of treatment was in the best interest of the patient. However, this practice opposes the principle of patient autonomy and undermines the ethical basis of surrogate decision making. At the same time, although Preference advocates endorsed the

> importance of the patient's values and priorities for decision making, it is not clear when and how they make these values and priorities known to the clinical team.

Lilley et al. propose early use of shared decision-making to address this problem. "By applying this model, surgeons and intensivists can play a pivotal role by advising surrogates early on that their primary responsibility is to focus on the patient's values and that the medical team will provide recommendations that are consistent with those values" [15].

Such early engagement is frequently missing from the decision-making process regarding surgical intervention in the critically ill patient. In a discourse analysis of electronic medical records of ICU patients, treatment focused specifically on physiology-centered interventions. Only when interventions failed to achieve physiologic goals did written explanations of a clinician's decision-making process turn to engagement with surrogates in treatment decisions. Notably, "the documentation focused on procedures and health states that patients and families wish to avoid, with little description of outcomes or events that patients and families were hoping for or would value." Indeed, the ubiquitous phrase "goals of care" was used by physicians in a largely negative context, as an expression of poor prognosis, a term to describe conflict between the care team and family, or the rationale to limit specific treatments, such as re-intubation or dialysis [16]. Again, the patient's values regarding an acceptable or desired outcome were not defined, suggesting that these preferences were not queried. As such, one cannot say that most medical care in the ICU is "preference-based" treatment or treatment formulated via shared decision-making.

9.7 Shared Decision-Making

Shared decision-making (SDM) has been defined as "an approach where clinicians and patients share the best available evidence when faced with the task of making decisions, and where patients are supported to consider options, to achieve informed preferences" [17]. However, SDM is a term frequently used and poorly understood, particularly among surgeons. In an international survey of 650 trauma and acute care surgeons, 74% of surgeons said they were familiar with the term "shared decision-making," but only 45% could provide a definition of SDM that correctly described the process of clinicians actively involving the patient in treatment decisions [18]. Instead, most surgeons defined SDM as a multidisciplinary care team that collaboratively made treatment plans for patients; the patient was not included in the definition at all. Furthermore, while surgeons acknowledged that "understanding the patient's preferences" was critical to SDM, "spending time to investigate about the patient's preferences" was considered one of the least relevant aspects of SDM. Indeed, time is a crucial factor to surgeons implementing shared decision-making tools in an emergency; "sometimes decisions are urgent and have to be made right away" was the most cited barrier to using SDM. In their analysis of survey responses, Cobianchi et al. conclude that trauma and acute care surgeons lack an understanding of shared decision-making and the benefits it can provide.

Perhaps the most effective and efficient shared decision-making tool, at least within the surgical profession, is the "Best Case/Worst Case" technique. Best Case/Worst Case consists of the following: The surgeon uses a pen and paper to draw a figurative representation of the treatment choices for the patient. Using lines, arrows, and stars, the surgeon compares two or more treatment choices and uses "narrative to tell a story about how the patient might experience the outcomes in the best and worst case scenarios." Surgeons use their own experience, as well as the objective data known about morbidity and mortality, to offer estimations of the most likely outcome based on that specific patient's clinical circumstance. Additionally, the surgeon takes time to explain how the treatment options may impact the patient's overall health, function, and independence. This information is thus no longer concealed from the patient due to the surgeon's concern that the patient (or their family) will be frightened or lose hope. Instead, the surgeon can acknowledge that medical-surgical treatments have limitations and thereby establish realistic expectations for various treatments.

At the end of the discussion, during which the patient is invited to engage, ask questions, and voice their own opinion on the acceptability of each treatment and its best and worst outcomes, the surgeon offers a treatment recommendation. In focus groups, both surgeons and patients "praised the tool for depicting both sides of the story;" patients specifically liked this tool because it "is an opportunity for patients to consider and incorporate personal values and goals when making a complex decision" [19].

The genius of "Best Case/Worst Case" is that it is adaptable to both acute and elective scenarios, and it honors patient preferences as well as the expertise of surgeons. It is straightforward, intuitive, and quick, allowing surgeons and patients (or surrogates) to dive deeply and immediately into the decision at hand and what is at stake with each treatment choice. It bucks the surgeon's instinctual fix-it modus operandi, where they see "the surgical disease as an isolated abnormality that can be 'fixed' through a surgery while failing to fully consider chronic debilitating conditions that cannot be cured through surgery" [7]. It allows the patient to consider the likelihood of survival and the quality of that future life, which is not at the forefront of a patient's mind when his or her body is under threat.

In essence, Best Case/Worst Case acknowledges that "life" has many nuanced definitions, and each treatment decision is, in many ways, as unique as the patient themselves. Best Case/Worst Case and other shared decision-making methods like it provide balanced consideration of a patient's values, a surgeon's clinical wisdom, and limitations of medicine's ability to sustain life but its ceaseless ability to care for a patient throughout life, especially at its end.

9.8 Conclusion

Ethics looks at "how well we respect those we encounter." Respect demands a person "to be artistic, subjective, freeing, reciprocal, gentle, engaged, holistic, attentive, patient, modest, trusting, graceful, reconciling, humanizing. But surgeons must be scientific, objective, detached. Therein lies the ethical complexity of patient encounters" [20]. Cassell observes similarly:

> Surgeons, unlike patients, know that caring about the patient is useless unless the surgeon possesses the technique, knowledge, and clinical judgment to care adequately for that patient… If the surgeon has the foundation, hands, knowledge, and clinical judgment then, and only then, can caring about the patient as a person improve results. Without these basic characteristics of a good surgeon, the top layer, caring is merely 'window dressing'. [21]

Sometimes, respecting or caring for the patient aligns comfortably with the objective evidence of the clinical scenario. I personally do not hesitate when recommending surgery to most patients with a history, exam, and CT confirming a diagnosis of acute appendicitis. The situation is harmonious, aligning the four ethical principles upon which medical ethics are founded—non-maleficence, beneficence, self-determination, and justice. I can rapidly alleviate a patient's suffering and restore their health in a way that is of minimal harm to them and cost-efficient. However, the critically ill patient with a surgical abdomen is different. The time pressure, the emotional intensity, the cost and resources involved, and the knowledge that suffering will be prolonged if not permanent for the patient can create a true ethical dilemma.

Ethical dilemmas and the deliberation needed to reach a resolution are necessarily collaborative and collective, drawing on multiple individual viewpoints. However, surgeons frequently work alone, with our decisions discussed collectively only in a post hoc fashion at a weekly Morbidity and Mortality Conference. The decision to operate is generally felt to be the surgeon's alone, which is why, in these critical moments, respect and caring for the patient are vital. Shared decision-making is that collaborative and collective process to reach an ethical decision regarding a patient's treatment. Instead of putting rationality and objectivity first, it must put care for the patient at the forefront of everything we do.

In my first month as an attending surgeon, I took care of a woman with cirrhosis and portal hypertension with a mesenteric venous thrombus. The blood clot was slowly reducing the oxygenated blood flow to her small intestine, and after two weeks of minimal improvement on anticoagulation and antibiotics, she became acutely ill. I immediately went into fix-it mode, notifying the OR and talking with the anesthesiologist. I paused and re-examined her labs and saw her platelets of 12,000 and bilirubin newly elevated to 4.5. I reviewed her CT scan and saw the minefield of caput medusa veins preventing a swift and efficient laparotomy incision. I went to her husband sheepishly and told him that surgery was not an option. He begged me to save his wife, blessing my hands with holy water from Lourdes while I said through tears, "I'm sorry, I can't, I can't."

Her husband and I were both realizing, at the same time but in different ways, that even the miracle of surgery has its limits.

I left the hospital that evening knowing that the patient would die. I thought about her husband and the anger and pain he must be feeling. I thought I had done a poor job caring for her, having failed to save her life and then having failed to shepherd her into life's final moments with peace. I regretted that last part most of all; it seemed as if I could have cared more.

A week later, I received an email from the patient's husband, telling me that his wife had died surrounded by family a few days after our interaction. He wrote to me to apologize for any hurt his words and actions may have caused; "I truly believe that you are a very good and caring person," he said. "As testimony of my true feelings, if I or any of my loved ones ever need surgical intervention, I will seek you out."

I was stunned by the graciousness and generosity of his words.

Joan Cassell writes, "caring cannot occur in a vacuum; it unfolds during the interaction between patient and surgeon. Caring is not something a surgeon does to a patient; it takes place between two unique human beings. Caring relationships are reciprocal and mutually reinforcing; trust elicits caring, which elicits trust" [22].

Perhaps this is why shared decision-making eases so much of the ethical stress of caring for the critically ill in need of an emergency operation. It places care at the center of all decisions. Just like a mother looking to understand the sadness of her child, or a man's thirst to know every thought held by his new lover, shared decision-making asks the surgeon to be curious about the qualities, beliefs, and values that make the patient in front of them a human, and not just a clinical problem to be sorted and fixed.

Acknowledgments I would like to acknowledge my father, John Bakke, MD, for his generous and thoughtful editing of early drafts of this chapter.

Competing Interests I have no competing interests or financial disclosures.

References

1. Wancata LM, Abdelsattar ZM, Suwanabol PA, Campbell DA, Hendren S. Outcomes after surgery for benign and malignant small bowel obstruction. J Gastrointest Surg. 2017;21(2):363–71.
2. Blair SL, Chu DZ, Schwarz RE. Outcome of palliative operations for malignant bowel obstruction in patients with peritoneal carcinomatosis from nongynecological cancer. Ann Surg Oncol. 2001;8(8):632–7.
3. Smith JW, Knight Davis J, Quatman-Yates CC, Waterman BL, Strassels SA, Wong JD, et al. Loss of community-dwelling status among survivors of high-acuity emergency general surgery disease. J Am Geriatr Soc. 2019;67(11):2289–97.
4. Kennedy CA, Shipway D, Barry K. Frailty and emergency abdominal surgery: a systematic review and meta-analysis. Surgeon. 2022;20(6):e307–14.
5. Briggs A, Handzel RM, Kutcher ME, Peitzman AB, Forsythe RM. Predisposed to failure? The challenge of rescue in the medical intensive care unit. J Trauma Acute Care Surg. 2019;87(4):774–81.

6. Huckaby LV, Dadashzadeh ER, Li S, Campwala I, Gabriel L, Sperry J, et al. Accuracy of risk estimation for surgeons versus risk calculators in emergency general surgery. J Surg Res. 2022;278:57–63.
7. Hornor M, Khan U, Cripps MW, Cook Chapman A, Knight-Davis J, Puzio TJ, et al. Futility in acute care surgery: first do no harm. Trauma Surg Acute Care Open. 2023;8(1):e001167.
8. Rousseau AF, Prescott HC, Brett SJ, Weiss B, Azoulay E, Creteur J, et al. Long-term outcomes after critical illness: recent insights. Crit Care. 2021;25(1):108.
9. Ho VP, Roach MJ, Berg KA, Deverakonda DL, Kanuika P, Arko B, et al. In their own words: recovery after emergency general surgery in the older patient. Trauma Surg Acute Care Open. 2023;8(1):e001138.
10. Moore F. Metabolic care of the surgical patient. 1st ed. Philadelphia: W. B. Saunders Company; 1959. p. vii.
11. Kulkarni SS, Briggs A, Sacks OA, Rosengart MR, White DB, Barnato AE, et al. Inner deliberations of surgeons treating critically-ill emergency general surgery patients: a qualitative analysis. Ann Surg. 2021;274(6):1081–8.
12. Cassell J. Expected miracles: surgeons at work. Philadelphia: Temple University Press; 1991. p. 49–50.
13. Fried TR, Bradley EH, Towle VR, Allore H. Understanding the treatment preferences of seriously ill patients. N Engl J Med. 2002;346(14):1061–6.
14. Sokas C, Yeh IM, Coogan K, Bernacki R, Mitchell S, Bader A, et al. Older adult perspectives on medical decision making and emergency general surgery: "It had to be done…". J Pain Symptom Manag. 2021;61(5):948–54.
15. Lilley EJ, Morris MA, Sadovnikoff N, Luxford JM, Changoor NR, Bystricky A, et al. "Taking over somebody's life": experiences of surrogate decision-makers in the surgical intensive care unit. Surgery. 2017;162(2):453–60.
16. Kruser JM, Benjamin BT, Gordon EJ, Michelson KN, Wunderink RG, Holl JL, et al. Patient and family engagement during treatment decisions in an ICU: a discourse analysis of the electronic health record. Crit Care Med. 2019;47(6):784–91.
17. Elwyn G, Frosch D, Thomson R, Joseph-Williams N, Lloyd A, Kinnersley P, et al. Shared decision making: a model for clinical practice. J Gen Intern Med. 2012;27(10):1361–7.
18. Cobianchi L, Dal Mas F, Agnoletti V, Ansaloni L, Biffl W, Butturini G, et al. Time for a paradigm shift in shared decision making in trauma and emergency surgery? Results from an international survey. World J Emerg Surg. 2023;18(1):14.
19. Kruser JM, Taylor LJ, Campbell TC, Zelenski A, Johnson SK, Nabozny MJ, et al. "Best case/worst case": training surgeons to use a novel communication tool for high-risk acute surgical problems. J Pain Symptom Manag. 2017;53(4):711–719.e5.
20. Brown D. Surgical ethics: theory and practice background. In: Ferreres AR, editor. Surgical ethics: principles and practice. 1st ed. Cham: Springer International Publishing; 2019. p. 28.
21. Cassell J. Expected miracles: surgeons at work. Philadelphia: Temple University Press; 1991. p. 28–30.
22. Cassell J. Expected miracles: surgeons at work. Philadelphia: Temple University Press; 1991. p. 215.

Chapter 10
Social Responsibility in Surgical Practice

Megan G. Janeway, Sheina Theodore, and Danby Kang

10.1 Introduction to Social Responsibility

We define social responsibility in medicine as the professional duty of physicians to improve the health of their society. This responsibility entails diagnosing the social causes of disparities in healthcare access and outcomes, both at the level of the individual patient and in the community, and providing both local and systemic interventions [1–3]. Social responsibility is multidimensional and involves political advocacy, community partnership, research, and education [4].

The purpose of this chapter is to explore the role of social responsibility in medicine and more specifically in surgical practice. The goal is to help practitioners understand what is meant by social responsibility and to encourage integration of the principles into individual and institutional surgical practices. We will discuss the relevance of social responsibility in the healthcare climate today, provide examples of how our profession is increasingly integrating social responsibility, and outline what social responsibility looks like in surgical practice.

10.2 Social Responsibility in Healthcare Today

Over the last 20 years, literature dedicated to healthcare disparities has grown, demonstrating now more than ever the need for greater recognition and incorporation of social responsibility in medicine. Two reports from 1974 (The Canadian Lalonde)

M. G. Janeway (✉) · S. Theodore · D. Kang
Division of Trauma and Acute Care Surgery, Department of Surgery, Boston Medical Center, Boston, MA, USA

Boston University Chobanian & Avedisian School of Medicine, Boston, MA, USA
e-mail: megan.janeway@bmc.org

F. Jotterand, C. Bosco (eds.), *Fostering Humanism in Surgery*, New Paradigms in Healthcare, https://doi.org/10.1007/978-3-031-82771-6_10

and 1980 (The Black Report in the United Kingdom) were central to defining socially determined health disparities and inspiring other nations to examine their own delivery of healthcare. Not until 1996 was the term "social determinants of health" used regularly and methodically. Four categories of etiology emerged: genetic and biological factors, medical care, individual health-related behaviors, and the "social characteristics within which living takes place [5]."

Literature over the last 10 years identified sources of health disparity across the United States. This research spanned all medical disciplines and allowed providers to better understand the cause-and-effect relationship. These causes are disparate and range from geographic barriers to care, social environment and support, healthcare provider cultural awareness, hospital and institutional forces, and the intersection between all of these. Regardless of the cause, the effect is the same—inequitable access and outcomes for those affected. To provide quality care and ensure equity, we should employ social responsibility and address these social determinants of health directly.

10.2.1 Patient and Social Factors: Race, Ethnicity, Gender, Sexual Orientation, and Socioeconomic Position

Key drivers of social determinants of health in the surgical patient population include race, ethnicity, gender, sexual orientation, and socioeconomic position. Race has been shown to be a significant factor in women eligible for hysterectomy: women who are African American, Hispanic, or Asian/Pacific Islander are less likely to receive minimally invasive hysterectomy compared to open abdominal hysterectomy [6]. As another example, in the non-white orthopedic population, immobility and mortality are higher compared to that of whites, and time to assess and treat black patients for hip fracture is significantly longer [7]. It has been well-established that these types of social determinants of health (SDH) impact surgical outcomes [8]. It is also well-established, but perhaps not as recognized, that reducing disparities will impact the upstream effects of SDH [9, 10]. Examples of disparities include large survival differences in breast cancer patients with low socioeconomic status among all races even when enrolled in Medicare and Medicaid [11]. Similarly, authors have noted decreased eligibility and access to bariatric surgery among those with medical indications but without private insurance, low income or low education, and non-white race [12]. These key patient and social drivers, and the impact they have on equity, should be better understood and addressed.

10.2.2 System Factors: Healthcare Access and Delivery

Hospital and insurance forces have also been implicated in contributing to healthcare disparities. The authors of a 2015 analysis of the potential impact of the Centers for Medicare and Medicaid policy, the Hospital Readmissions Reduction Program, noted that minority-serving hospitals disproportionately incurred more penalties and severe reductions in reimbursement [13]. The ability to access and deliver healthcare is also impacted by geography. Living in a rural environment and the distance to tertiary-level care both contribute to health disparities [14]. A more recent study, as part of the American College of Surgeons' collaborative toward reducing disparities in surgical care, proposes a new conceptual model of surgical access disparities. This model includes provider access, surgical indication detection, progression to surgery, and receipt of optimal care, with each category sequentially influencing the other categories [15].

10.2.3 Provider-Related Factors

Several provider-specific factors have been shown to contribute, either indirectly or directly, to disparate healthcare. Studies have shown that implicit bias of physicians may negatively impact patient communication and clinical assessments [16–19]. Providers may feel uncomfortable or unprepared to address social risk factors [20]. Literature has suggested that lack of provider education contributes to healthcare disparities among minority and underserved populations [21–23].

10.3 Challenges for Surgeons

The topic of social responsibility in medicine is controversial. We would be remiss not to address the real challenges that remain in the practical application of social responsibility in surgery. Many have taken the position that physicians should focus their responsibilities to individual patients and that their responsibilities to society are limited [24, 25]. Is it reasonable or feasible to mandate surgeons engage in the idea of social responsibility without the support from their peers or from employers, healthcare corporations, or academic institutions? Is it reasonable or feasible without training and education? Is it reasonable or feasible without financial support from their institution or professional organizations? Without the appropriate resources and support provided, surgeons are unlikely to be successful in their engagement, and this may result in learned helplessness, which negatively impacts the patient. Surgeons already struggle with limited time, limited reimbursement, and limited academic advancement incentives for activities outside of Relative Value Units (RVU—a measure of value used in the reimbursement formula for physician services generation). Thus, we must not only show the importance of this work for patient outcomes but also propose ways to change the system so that incorporating social responsibility into practice has tangible benefits. Therefore, when discussing this topic, individual and systematic efforts will be described in addition to individual and systemic benefits.

10.4 Incorporating Social Responsibility into Surgical Practice

10.4.1 Education and Training

In addition to more investigation geared to improving the health of our patients as we consider social determinants and risk factors, we also need an emphasis on social responsibility in surgical training and requirements that promote action, such as advocacy training. Medical students now learn not only about social determinants of health but how these factors are the major drivers of health. Medical school curricula and continuing medical education targeting background knowledge of the social determinants of health would help lay a contextualized background for all care teams at an institution. Many interns and residents are now coming into their training with a broader perspective of healthcare: their view is more socially conscious. Thinking more about communities and populations—on a local, national, and global scale—is intuitive. We need to ensure that volunteerism and commitment to social change do not decline during clinical training [26]. Recently, a REVOLUTIONS framework was proposed to have socially accountable medical education [27]. Although this work focuses more on undergraduate medical education, it can be used as a guide for surgical educators as we look to incorporate new approaches within our training programs that are innovative, collaborative, participatory, and transformative [28].

In addition to broadening our residency curriculums, faculty need to show residents that there is mentorship regarding the social determinants of health in relation to surgical patients.

Surgeons ought to demonstrate that advocacy is a foundation of professionalism in medicine. A 2016 Institute of Medicine report concluded, "To impact health equity… requires more than just accruing knowledge, health professionals must develop appropriate skills and attitudes to be advocates for change [29]." These skills can be taught to medical students and residents and should continue throughout a surgeon's career to nurture our teams in socially acceptable practices. Ideally this will then increase trainee interest in health equity and service in a cycle that will continue to perpetuate itself until these inequities are resolved.

10.4.2 Professional Leadership and Governing Bodies

Surgical professional associations and governing bodies have a responsibility to encourage practicing surgeons and healthcare teams to incorporate socially responsible behaviors in their daily practice. Multiple professional societies have proclaimed edicts describing a physician's responsibility toward the whole health of their patients. The ACGME specifically developed general competencies that address the "development of core professional attributes, such as altruism and social accountability, needed to provide effective care in a multidimensionally diverse society." The identified aim is to prepare future physicians to be "responsive to the needs of patients and society that supersede self-interest [30]. Similarly, the American Medical Association's Code of Medical Ethics specifies that "...each physician has an obligation to share in providing care to the indigent... All physicians should work to ensure that the needs of the poor in their communities are met... Caring for the poor should be a regular part of the physician's practice schedule" [31]. Finally, the Association of American Medical Colleges Core Curriculum Working Group states that residents "must use their influence to improve the health of the communities where they live and practice," and they must "understand the roles that physicians can play in meeting the healthcare needs of the poor, in addressing health inequities that exist between different populations in the society, and in promoting the general health of the public" [32].

Given these professional edicts, institutions have a responsibility to encourage practicing surgeons and healthcare teams to incorporate behaviors supporting those edicts in their daily practice. Additional mandates in surgical training, such as a minimum number of didactic hours in residency or CME credits devoted to teaching about socially responsible practice, may be helpful and are currently the practice of some graduate medical education programs [33–35]. Continuing medical education targeting background knowledge of the social determinants of health would help lay a contextualized background for all care teams at an institution. As we move past a focus on standard surgical outcomes to patient-centered outcomes and shared decision processes, it is imperative surgeons understand the nuances of our diverse patients and their needs.

10.4.3 Current National Opportunities for Engagement

Broadening the surgical community's support for incorporating social responsibility into surgery requires the investment of our national organizations from the top and grassroots movements on the ground. There are some examples of how the surgical community is currently promoting and achieving social responsibility in surgery:

1. Socially Responsible Surgery is an organization founded in 2014 with a mission of establishing social responsibility as a core value of surgical practice. This

group has chapters at many surgical programs across the United States and uses four pillars—research, education, advocacy, and service—to foster engagement for advocacy and surgical equity [36, 37].
2. The American College of Surgeons (ACS) Committee on Trauma working group, ISAVE, Improving Social Determinants of Health to Attenuate Violence, proposes strategies for trauma centers to address root causes of violence [38]. Current projects from this group include incorporating social and trauma-informed care into all trauma centers and promoting hospital investment in marginalized communities to reduce firearm violence.
3. The ACS Committee on Health Care Disparities works to address the irrefutable association between the incidence of and outcomes from a host of surgical diseases and the many barriers to access to care [39].
4. The Association of Surgical Education (ASE) runs a Committee on Citizenship and Global Responsibility which supports outreach projects performing or teaching surgery in countries/areas where resources are scarce [40].

10.4.4 Academic Practice and Scholarly Research

Taking a scholarly approach to advocacy by encouraging and participating in research that contributes to a better understanding of socioeconomic factors and effective interventions to address them is critically important to improving surgical care [6]. Surgeons must push past simply publishing on disparities and translate this academic information into action for our patients and our communities. Surgeons should seek to understand how SDH affects their patients, using patient-centered research to understand from patients how these affect their interaction with the healthcare system. The time has passed for gathering data and "pointing it out." Now research should be undertaken to understand the issue and propose and test a solution [41]. Surgeons can engage in this work by enhancing their research methodologies to an intervention-based approach, such as small scalable interventions and direct advocacy work.

10.4.5 Incorporate Social Responsibility into Individual and Daily Clinical Practice

Social responsibility can and must be integrated into everyday surgical practice. Failure to address the underlying causes of disease and ill-health risks perpetuating a cycle of inequity, disparity, and inequality that will remain for generations to come. While many surgeons may see this outside of their scope of practice, it is essential to understand and address the importance of the effect social determinants have on health outcomes, as they are often modifiable risk factors and have a strong influence on health outcomes [42]. We suggest several essential components that can be implemented to ensure socially responsible surgical practice.

10.4.6 Knowing and Addressing Patients' Social Determinants of Health

The first step in socially responsible practice is to screen patients for social risk factors. There are many validated social determinant of health-screening tools available to identify patient needs [43]. Physicians and care teams should be able to identify food insecurity, interpersonal violence, unsafe housing, language barriers, substance use disorders, and other key social determinants of health to fully understand the patient experience. Identifying and responding to factors outside the clinical encounter that influence health can lead to significant improvements in a patient's overall health [44]. The patient's family may also benefit if risk factors like food insecurity and housing are addressed.

Providers and hospitals need to prioritize gathering SDH data during a clinical encounter. Gathering and analyzing local patient data can help providers better understand the population they care for and tailor to patient needs. Clinicians, clinical leaders, and hospital executives from across the country agree that using SDH data in patient care can improve outcomes and the patient experience [45]. In fact, some hospitals have started collecting this data on all patients routinely and have shown improved social services utilization by patients with SDH needs [46, 47]. When SDH data is obtained and reviewed, patient needs can be identified and acted upon. Interventions such as medical respite centers, robust case management programs, wraparound services, and investments in affordable housing are cost-effective, can reduce acute care utilization rates, and reduce readmissions [48–50]. In addition to consistent, widespread data collection and analysis, we recommend expansion of social services to allow for better access by patients to address risk factors any time they are identified.

10.4.7 Advocating for Patients

Identifying and becoming involved in advocacy activities that relate not only to surgery but also the issues that affect the long-term health of our patients and our community is essential. Community engagement leads to a better understanding of the issues facing patients, and advocacy training will enable providers to be more proactive in addressing the root causes of surgical inequity and healthcare disparities [51]. Furthermore, collaboration with other medical specialties that do excellent work addressing social risk factors and inequities, such as pediatrics or family medicine, on both educational and clinical initiatives may be beneficial. For example, the American Academy of Family Physicians released a position paper outlining specific policies that will address these upstream health determinants, such as guaranteeing population-level access to healthcare, anti-poverty programs, civil rights, and anti-discrimination [52]. Obstetricians routinely partake in advocacy for reproductive rights, and pediatricians have developed many innovative grassroots initiatives to address the social needs of families that may affect the health of children, such as free tax help in clinics and literacy efforts [53, 54]. Surgeons need to be on the forefront of advocacy and understand the power they wield to shape policy recommendations to educate legislators on healthcare.

Advocating at the individual patient level can include leveraging community resources for patients. Surgeons have a great deal of agency and power, and our voices can be used for change. Getting surgeons involved early in advocacy at the hospital, state, and national levels will help us improve access to care for our patients. Advocacy training and community engagement will help surgeons take a step across this low barrier to increase involvement in advocacy on behalf of our patients. We as surgeons ought to use our power and privilege to stand up for our patients.

10.5 Conclusions

Surgeons and surgical care teams must be able to identify key social risk factors to fully understand the patient experience. Screening for these social risk factors must be incorporated and standardized into the care of all patients, and care teams must follow through to provide linkages to community services. Surgeons ought to utilize research not solely for publication but to better understand the socioeconomic factors impacting patients and communities and to effect change through intervention or advocacy. Addressing SDH through social responsibility is of critical importance for improving the care we provide [4].

We must understand our patient's social determinants of health; they are as important as their genetic risk factors. We cannot provide comprehensive care without understanding the unique needs of our patients and communities and we can use our position to influence those who hold the power to impact those communities. We need to use research—not just to point out disparities but to translate this into action through local change or advocacy. We need to stop being silent on injustices, both big and small, and use our voices as healthcare workers to improve care for our patients.

More needs to be done to ensure that we not only deliver excellent healthcare but that we do it in an equitable and sustainable way. There are continued challenges that we can work to address, such as getting support from our institutions and finding ways to incentivize time dedicated to addressing our patient's needs. As surgeons, we must aim for innovative programs and curricula to both train surgeons in social responsibility and raise the bar in the delivery of better and more equitable care.

References

1. Faulkner LR, McCurdy RL. Teaching medical students social responsibility: the right thing to do. Acad Med. 2000;75(4):346–50.
2. Bruhn JG. On social responsibility. J Med Educ. 1971;46(2):166–8.
3. Ferdinand DP, Nedunchezhian S, Ferdinand KC. Hypertension in African Americans: advances in community outreach and public health approaches. Prog Cardiovasc Dis. 2020;63(1):40–5.
4. Dharamsi S, Ho A, Spadafora SM, Woollard R. The physician as health advocate: translating the quest for social responsibility into medical education and practice. Acad Med 2011;86(9):1108–1113.
5. World Health Organization. Action on the social determinants of health: learning from previous experiences. Geneva: World Health Organization; 2010. http://www.who.int/social_determinants/corner/SDHDP1.pdf. Accessed 11 Apr 2024.
6. Pollack LM, Olsen MA, Gehlert SJ, Chang SH, Lowder JL. Racial/ethnic disparities/differences in hysterectomy route in women likely eligible for minimally invasive surgery. J Minim Invasive Gynecol. 2020;27(5):1167–1177.e2. http://www.sciencedirect.com/science/article/pii/S1553465019304108. Accessed 11 Apr 2024.
7. Frier A, Barnett F, Devine S, Barker R. Understanding disability and the 'social determinants of health': how does disability affect peoples' social determinants of health? Disabil Rehabil. 2018;40(5):538–47.
8. Janeway M, Wilson S, Sanchez SE, Arora TK, Dechert T. Citizenship and social responsibility in surgery: a review. JAMA Surg. 2022;157(6):532–9.
9. Braveman PA, Egerter SA, Mockenhaupt RE. Broadening the focus: the need to address the social determinants of health. Am J of Prev Med. 2011;40(1):S4–S18.
10. Williams DR, Costa MV, Odunlami AO, Mohammed SA. Moving upstream: how interventions that address the social determinants of health can improve health and reduce disparities. JPHMP. 2008;14(6):S8–S17.
11. Silber JH, Rosenbaum PR, Ross RN, Reiter JG, Niknam BA, Hill AS, et al. Disparities in breast cancer survival by socioeconomic status despite medicare and medicaid insurance. Milbank Q. 2018;96(4):706–54.
12. Martin M, Beekley A, Kjorstad R, Sebesta J. Socioeconomic disparities in eligibility and access to bariatric surgery: a national population-based analysis. Surg Obes Relat Dis. 2010;6(1):8–15.
13. Shih T, Ryan AM, Gonzalez AA, Dimick JB. Medicare's hospital readmission reduction program in surgery may disproportionately affect minority-serving hospitals. Ann Surg. 2015;261(6):1027–31.
14. RRH: rural and remote health article: 5147 – geographic disparities associated with travel to medical care and attendance in programs to prevent/manage chronic illness among middle-aged and older adults in Texas. https://www.rrh.org.au/journal/article/5147. Accessed 11 Apr 2024.
15. de Jager E, Levine A, Udyavar NR, Burstin HR, Bhulani N, Hoyt DB, et al. Disparities in surgical access: a systematic literature review, conceptual model, and evidence map. J Am Coll Surg. 2019;228(3):276–98.
16. Green AR, Carney DR, Pallin DJ, Ngo LH, Raymond KL, Iezzoni LI, et al. Implicit bias among physicians and its prediction of thrombolysis decisions for black and white patients. J Gen Intern Med. 2007;22(9):1231–8.
17. Sabin JA, Rivara FP, Greenwald AG. Physician implicit attitudes and stereotypes about race and quality of medical care. Med Care. 2008;46(7):678–85.
18. Tamayo-Sarver JH, Dawson NV, Hinze SW, Cydulka RK, Wigton RS, Albert JM, et al. The effect of race/ethnicity and desirable social characteristics on physicians' decisions to prescribe opioid analgesics. Acad Emerg Med. 2003;10(11):1239–48.
19. Sabin JA, Riskind RG, Nosek BA. Health care providers' implicit and explicit attitudes toward lesbian women and gay men. Am J Public Health. 2015;105(9):1831–41.

20. Makadon HJ. Ending LGBT invisibility in health care: the first step in ensuring equitable care. Cleve Clin J Med. 2011;78(4):220–4.
21. Kattari SK, Bakko M, Hecht HK, Kattari L. Correlations between healthcare provider interactions and mental health among transgender and nonbinary adults. SSM Popul Health. 2019;10 https://doi.org/10.1016/j.ssmph.2019.100525.
22. Prokup JA, Andridge R, Havercamp SM, Yang EA. Health care disparities of Ohioans with developmental disabilities across the lifespan. Ann Fam Med. 2017;15(5):471–4.
23. Bradley LJ, Clem J, Godsil R, MacFarlane J, Foster PP. Racial anxiety among medical residents: institutional implications of social accountability. J Health Care Poor Underserved. 2019;30(4S):105–15.
24. Huddle TS. Perspective: medical professionalism and medical education should not involve commitments to political advocacy. Acad Med. 2011;86(3):378–83. https://doi.org/10.1097/ACM.0b013e3182086efe.
25. Satel S. PC, how political correctness is corrupting medicine. New York: Perseus Books Group; 2002.
26. Grande D, Armstrong K. Community volunteerism of US physicians. J Gen Intern Med. 2008;23(12):1987–91. https://doi.org/10.1007/s11606-008-0811-x.1987-1991.
27. Ventres W, Dharamsi S. Socially accountable medical education – the REVOLUTIONS framework. Acad Med. 2015;90(12):1728.
28. Paprock KE, Mezirow J. Transformative dimensions of adult learning. Adult Educ Q. 1992;42(3):195–7. https://doi.org/10.1177/074171369204200309.
29. National Academies of Sciences E. A framework for educating health professionals to address the social determinants of health. 2016. https://www.nap.edu/catalog/21923/a-framework-for-educating-health-professionals-to-address-the-social-determinants-of-health. Accessed 11 Apr 2024.
30. ACGME policies and procedures. 2024. https://www.acgme.org/Portals/0/PDFs/ab_ACGMEPoliciesProcedures.pdf. Accessed 11 Apr 2024.
31. Code of Medical Ethics overview. American Medical Association. https://www.ama-assn.org/delivering-care/ethics/code-medical-ethics-overview. Accessed 11 Apr 2024.
32. Graduate Medical Education Core Curriculum. Association of American Medical Colleges [AAMC]. Core Curriculum Working Group (Group on Educational Affairs/Section for Graduate Medical Education. 2000. https://repository.library.georgetown.edu/handle/10822/930527. Accessed 11 Apr 2024.
33. Janeway MG, Lee SY, Caron E, Sausjord IK, Allee L, Sanchez SE, Dechert TA. Surgery service learning in preclinical years improves medical student attitudes toward surgery, clinical confidence, and social determinants of health screening. Am J Surg. 2020;219(2):346–54.
34. Medlock M, Weissman A, Wong SS, Carlo A, Zeng M, Borba C, et al. Racism as a unique social determinant of mental health: development of a didactic curriculum for psychiatry residents. MedEdPORTAL. 2017;13:10618.
35. Gard LA, Peterson J, Miller C, Ghosh N, Youmans Q, Didwania A, et al. Social determinants of health training in U.S. primary care residency programs: a scoping review. Acad Med. 2019;94(1):135–43.
36. Robinson TD, Oliveira TM, Timmes TR, Mills JM, Starr N, Fleming M, et al. Socially responsible surgery: building recognition and coalition. Front Surg. 2017;4:11.
37. Socially Responsible Surgery. https://www.sociallyresponsiblesurgery.org. Accessed 11 Apr 2024.
38. Dicker RA, Thomas A, Bulger EM, Stewart RM, Bonne S, Dechert TA, et al. Strategies for trauma centers to address the root causes of violence: recommendations from the Improving Social Determinants to Attenuate Violence (ISAVE) Workgroup of the American College of Surgeons Committee on Trauma. J Am Coll Surg. 2021;233(3):471–8.
39. American College of Surgeons Committee on Healthcare Disparities. https://www.facs.org/about-acs/governance/acs-committees/committee/573. Accessed 15 Apr 2024.

40. Association for Surgical Education—Standing Committees. https://www.surgicaleducation.com. Accessed 30 May 2024.
41. Bonner SN, Powell CA, Stewart JW, Dossett LA. Surgical care for racial and ethnic minorities and interventions to address inequities: a narrative review. Ann Surg. 2023;278(2):184–92.
42. Gómez CA, Kleinman DV, Pronk N, Wrenn Gordon GL, Ochiai E, Blakey C, et al. Addressing health equity and social determinants of health through healthy people 2030. J Public Health Manag Pract. 2021;27(Suppl 6):S249–57.
43. Buitron de la Vega P, Losi S, Sprague Martinez L, Bovell-Ammon A, Garg A, James T, et al. Implementing an EHR-based screening and referral system to address social determinants of health in primary care. Med Care. 2019;57:S133.
44. Williams DR, Costa MV, Odunlami AO, Mohammed SA. Moving upstream: how interventions that address the social determinants of health can improve health and reduce disparities. J Public Health Manag Pract. 2008;14(Suppl(Suppl)):S8–17.
45. Eisenson H, Mohta NS. Health care organizations can and must incorporate social determinants. NEJM Catalyst. 2020;1(3) https://doi.org/10.1056/CAT.20.0130.
46. Buitron de la Vega P, Losi S, Sprague Martinez L, Bovell-Ammon A, Garg A, James T, et al. Implementing an EHR-based screening and referral system to address social determinants of health in primary care. Med Care. 2019;57(Suppl 6 Suppl 2):S133–9.
47. Boston Medical Center. Health equity accelerator. www.bmc.org/health-equity-accelerator. Accessed 15 Apr 2024.
48. Kuehn BM. Hospitals turn to housing to help homeless patients. JAMA. 2019;321(9):822.
49. Bailey KT, Cook JT, Ettinger De Cuba S, Casey PH, Chilton M, Coleman SM, et al. Development of an index of subsidized housing availability and its relationship to housing insecurity. Hous Policy Debate. 2016;26(1):172–87.
50. Bailey P. Housing and health partners can work together to close the housing affordability gap. Center on Budget and Policy Priorities. 2020. https://www.cbpp.org/research/housing/housing-and-health-partners-can-work-together-to-close-the-housing-affordability. Accessed 15 Apr 2024.
51. Croft D, Jay SJ, Meslin EM, Gaffney MM, Odell JD. Perspective: is it time for advocacy training in medical education? Acad Med. 2012;87(9):1165–70.
52. Advancing health equity by addressing the social determinants of health in family medicine (position paper). American Academy of Family Physicians. 2019. https://www.aafp.org/about/policies/all/social-determinants-health-family-medicine.html. Accessed 14 Apr 2024.
53. Finkbeiner C, Doria C, Ellis-Kahana J, Loder CM. Changing obstetrics and gynecology residency education to combat reproductive injustice: a call to action. Obstet Gynecol. 2021;137(4):717–22.
54. Marcil LE, Hole MK, Wenren LM, Schuler MS, Zuckerman BS, Vinci RJ. Free tax services in pediatric clinics. Pediatrics. 2018;141(6):e20173608.

MIX
Papier aus verantwortungsvollen Quellen
Paper from responsible sources
FSC® C105338

If you have any concerns about our products,
you can contact us on
ProductSafety@springernature.com

In case Publisher is established outside the EU,
the EU authorized representative is:
Springer Nature Customer Service Center GmbH
Europaplatz 3, 69115 Heidelberg, Germany

Printed by Libri Plureos GmbH
in Hamburg, Germany